FROM BULLSHIT TO BOTOX

FROM BULLSHIT TO BOTOX

A REBEL'S GUIDE TO SELF-LOVE AND ETERNAL YOUTH

SANDRA LENA SILVERMAN

WITH CO-AUTHOR ERICA FLORENTINE
NEW YORK TIMES BEST SELLING AUTHOR

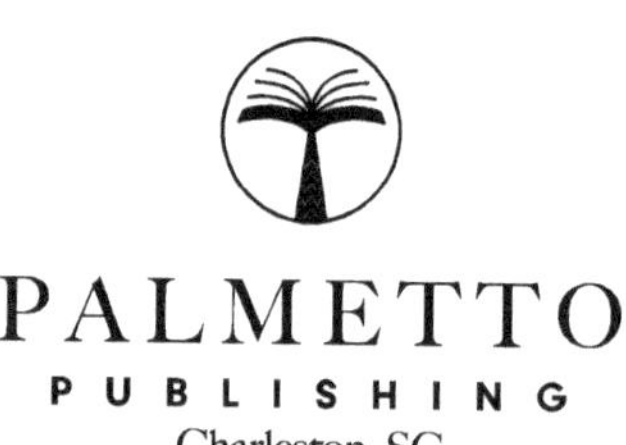

PALMETTO
PUBLISHING
Charleston, SC
www.PalmettoPublishing.com

Hardcover ISBN: 9798822951020
Paperback ISBN: 9798822951037
eBook ISBN: 9798822961029

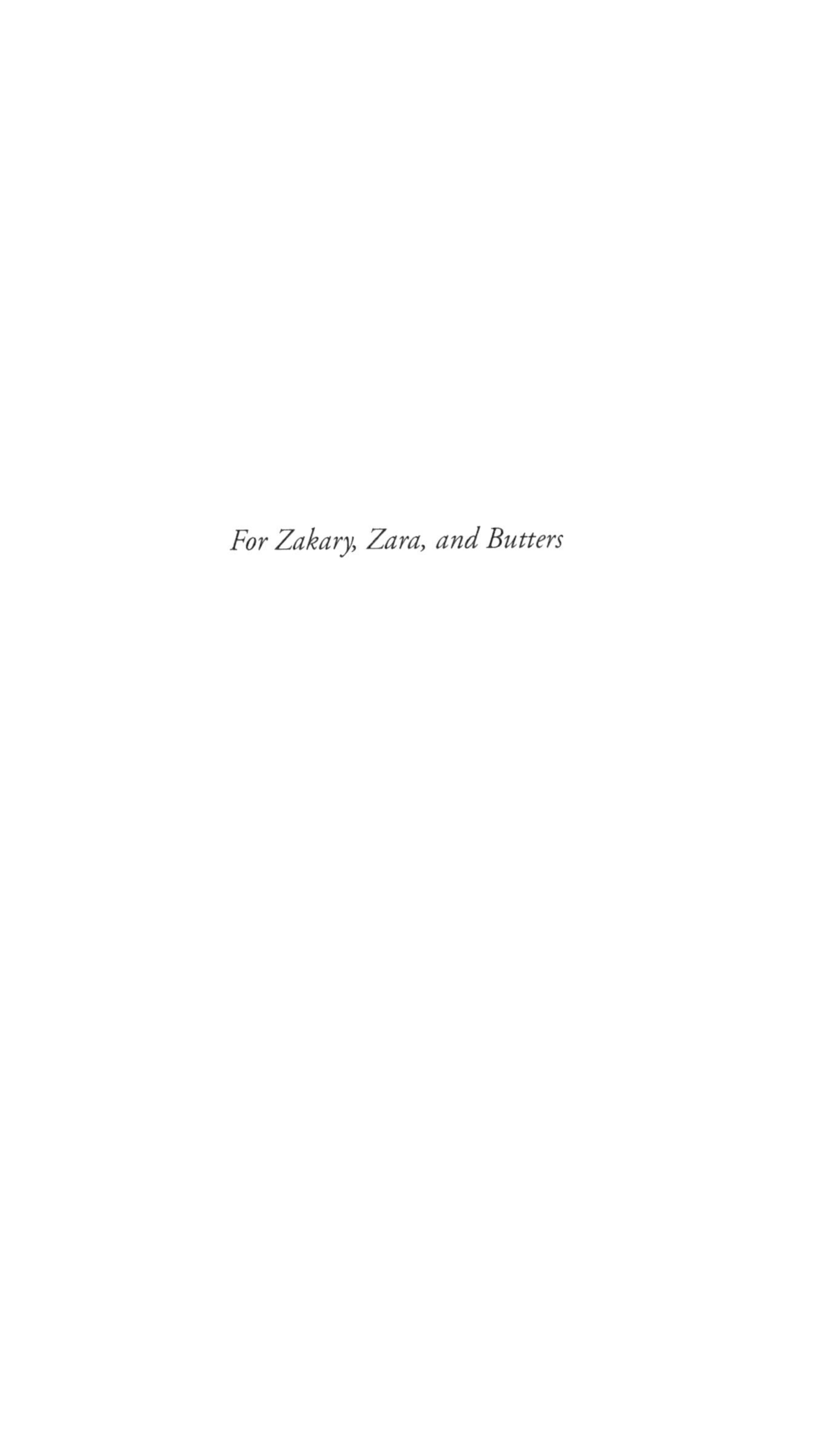
For Zakary, Zara, and Butters

TABLE OF CONTENTS

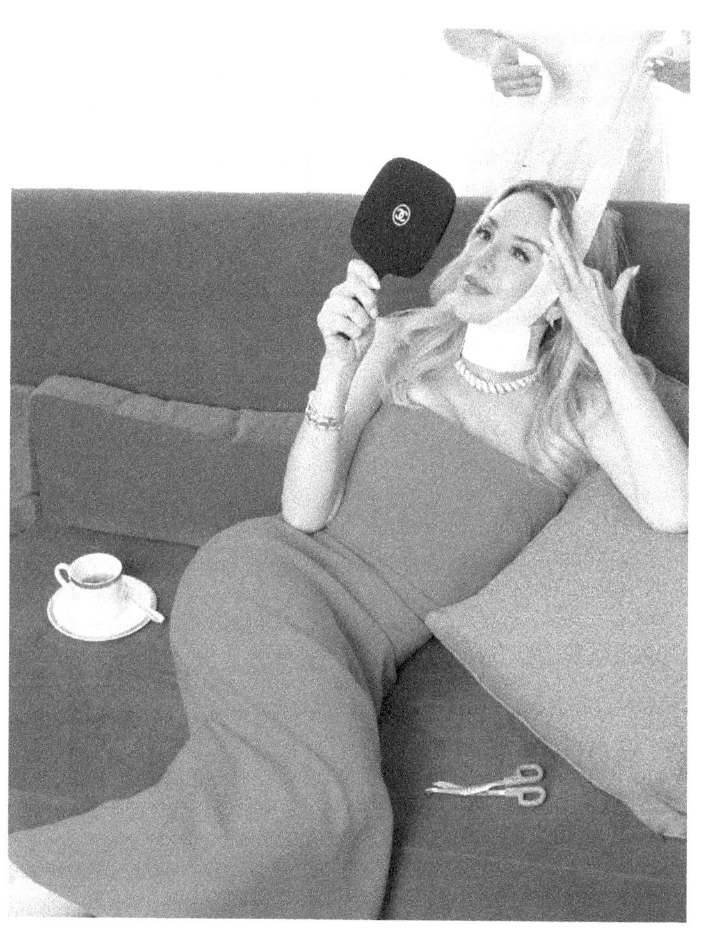

INTRODUCTION

Hello! My name is Sandra Lena Silverman (but my friends all call me Sandy!). The secret I would like to share with you all today is that I am fifty-three years old. The good news? Most people think I'm thirty-nine!

It's true that I look pretty good "for my age." However, it wasn't always this way. To be honest, my forties were an absolute, complete disaster. I went from looking good in my twenties and thirties, to being completely unrecognizable in my forties. I feel like I almost aged overnight, like maybe a pear, or one of those tubs of raspberries from Trader Joes that go moldy the minute you pick them up off the shelf. I'm sure I looked *fine* to everyone else, but when I looked in the mirror, I felt like I was staring at an old crone, a total Disney witch.

And I certainly didn't *feel* fine. I felt hideous. It was actually a sad state of affairs. My confidence was shattered, my marriage—which already had its share of ups and downs over the years—hit the rocks because I wasn't acting like myself, and my social life even petered out. I wanted the old Sandy back, the one who was fit and confident. Look, I know life isn't all about looks. That there are many major problems in this world, and even with this patriarchal society that makes us women feel like we need to be hot and skinny all the time. But I can't help it—I have my vanities, and if you've picked up this book, chances are you also have your vanities and want to look good. No shame in the game, sister. Also, someone needs to keep the trillion-dollar beauty industry afloat; we don't want the economy to collapse just because we've decided to embrace our grays. (Confession: I have never, and probably will never embrace my grays. It looks hot on a lot of women, especially those skinny and chic Parisians, but I am not one of them.)

Yes, I'd started plenty of preemptive measures leading up to my forties. I'd amped up my skincare routine, got into facials, peels, lasers, and other skin treatments, dabbled with Botox and filler, and had a few surgeries (breast implants and rhinoplasty in my twenties and a vaginal reconstruction in my late thirties—prompted by a health scare, which I'll get to). On the fitness end, I'd been working out pretty regularly since I'd met my husband in my late twenties. (I'll never forget one of the first conversations we ever had, this man told me I was *soft* and needed to get to the gym—what an asshole!) But my forties is really when I began to hate that stranger looking back at me in the mirror. *Is it all downhill from here?* I'd wonder.

Luckily, the answer has been a resounding, "NO!" In fact, it seems to only be getting better!

When I decided I really couldn't stand the way I was aging anymore, I invested in reversing time with the help of some additional modern medical practices. (Read: Plastic surgery.) I had a few more procedures and treatments in my forties to see if that would help me feel and look like my old self again. I got a mini tummy tuck, a facelift, face threads, and a breast lift with an implant swap. I got more regular about Botox (and then eventually switched to Dysport), and fillers, of course, and started getting them *everywhere*. I also got my teeth totally redone, including gum surgery, and I was also constantly injecting myself with peptides. (See, I told you I have tried a few things!)

Even after all of those efforts, things just weren't coming together fully like I'd hoped. It was very frustrating, considering the money and time I'd put into it. But after some trial and error—and plenty more nips and tucks—I realized I wasn't looking at the big picture. It turns out, it takes a lot more than just cutting or injecting your skin to look and feel amazing again. (Although it DEFI-NITELY helps. Stay with me here.)

This was when the health and wellness part of my journey started. It was the middle of March 2020, and the world was suddenly locked down in quarantine because of the COVID-19 pandemic. I was forty-nine years old. Each time I looked in the mirror or hopped on a Facetime call with friends, I thought, *Is this it? Is this the best that I'm ever going to look again? Even after ALL that stuff I did to myself, and all the money I spent?* The answer was, *Absolutely not!* While most people were watching Netflix or learning how to bake sourdough bread, I decided to be productive and figure out how to truly "reverse my age." And that, my friends, is when I started to look *hot*. But it wasn't just that I thought I looked good—everyone around me was noticing as well.

I'd really stepped it up. The first thing that helped was that I started working out daily. Yes, daily. (Come on, don't throw this book away at this point. I'm not here to say you need to work out for an hour every day, this is just how I kickstarted the wellness leg of my journey.) Also, it was lockdown and I had nothing else to do. I was lucky that my personal trainer Vanessa Reggiardo lived close to my house, so we began to consistently fitness train in my yard with a focus on weights. This wasn't new for me. I'd started to exercise regularly in my late twenties and I was an early adopter of weight training. But making sure I didn't miss a workout was crucial to seeing some serious changes in my body (later in this book I will explain what Vanessa and I did—and still do—during our weight training sessions).

After our hour-long workouts, Vanessa and I started to create our own lymphatic drainage protocols, which was nothing other than using tools (including fingers and a device called a FasciaBlaster) to help move fluids away from specific areas of my body. If you've ever used a Gua Sha stone on your face, you'll understand what I'm talking about—we used repetitive pressure to get the fluids moving. It took us some time, but we perfected a system that really worked. Soon I began to see all of the puffiness in my body disappear. It was a miracle. Everything became so clear. The mini tummy tuck I'd gotten wasn't a complete waste, because I could start to see my abs. The facelift that I'd had done turned out to be great as all the inflammation in my cheeks and under my eyes started to go away. I was starting to look sculpted, and even more lifted than I'd been in my thirties.

I also learned how important it is to be mindful of the food I put into my body (counting calories is by far the best way to lose and manage weight, which we'll get to!). The result was I finally lost those stubborn 10 pounds (for good!). It became incredibly obvious to me how important it is to be CON-SISTENT. And I mean consistent with *everything*—from treatments and procedures to all of my health and fitness practices. Consistency was the only way to see progress and then to maintain it.

Oh, and another huge win… because we were pretty much away from the world, I realized that I had tons of toxic people in my life who were constantly draining me, and that was showing up on my face. I committed to setting boundaries and saw a huge change in my overall happiness. With all these things in play, I looked fresh and youthful again. And like I said, it didn't go unnoticed.

Once we were out of the strictest lockdown and my friends started venturing out of their homes and into social situations again, people couldn't stop coming up to me and raving about the improvements I'd made to my face and body. I'm talking about women who enjoy a certain level of wealth—*Real Housewives of Miami* types who are no strangers to things like Botox and fillers and mini lifts and deep plane lifts and trying to look their best despite that annoying thing called gravity, which is so determined to bring us down—literally and figuratively.

"Oh my God, Sandy, *how* do you look so amazing?" they'd ask. "What's your secret? What work have you had done? Who did you go to? What was the procedure like? Was recovery painful? How much did it cost? What's your diet? What's your workout? Who's your stylist? Who's your dentist? What do I need to have done to look ten years younger too? Help me, Sandy, help me! Be my face, plastic surgery, and body guru!!!!!"

After a while, I started to get sick of all the questions. (Not the compliments. Those felt amazing. No one will ever get sick of compliments.) But it was too much to explain. So, one day, when I was at home enjoying the gorgeous outcome of my latest knee threading procedure (I'll write about that procedure a few chapters in), it dawned on me: I could actually just write ALL of this down. Everyone I know seems to be so secretive about what they've had done, but I have no secrets! I could explain in detail exactly what I did, how well it worked, what it cost, the pain and side effects, and everything and anything that people need to know about reversing your age. I would talk to experts to explain exactly what happens during procedures and I'd give my honest take on whether those procedures are worth it. I'd also talk about the procedures to *avoid*. I could basically write the "Official Plastic Surgery Handbook" for anyone who was contemplating these various procedures and wanted to hear the real story from someone who had actually tried it all.

I'd also get into what I do to *feel* younger, inside and out. That includes the workouts but also my internal wellness routine, what I do for my mental health (my life coach and psychic have both been SAVIORS), and the tips I've learned from my stylist on how to dress younger (but doing so tastefully—no one needs to see a woman in her fifties wearing a micro-mini bandeau dress!). To feel younger, I've tried it all too (*ahem*…ibogaine for anxiety!).

And when I say I've tried it all to look and feel younger, I'm not kidding. In fact, I've touched everywhere on my body except my left foot (I have a tattoo on my right foot). I already mentioned the breast implants, rhinoplasty, breast lift, injectables, vaginal reconstruction, face lift, mini tummy tuck, veneers and gum surgery, and peptide injections. But I've also done body sculpting and liposuction. An elbow lift. CO2 laser. Broad Band Light (BBL) laser. Chemical peels. Hair and eyelash extensions. Microblading. Testosterone. Vitamin injections. NAD injections. Neck Botox. Knee filler. Lymphatic treatment. Microneedling. Plant-based drugs. Therapeutic work. Biohacking tests and supplements. Diets and workout routines. Connective tissue work. ALL OF IT. (And so much more!)

You may have read that last paragraph with your jaw hanging on the ground. Or maybe you're shaking your head thinking, *Hah, there's no way this woman looks natural with all that work! She has to be over-tweaked!* But, if you're expecting me to look like some version of present-day Donatella Versace or someone who belongs on the TV show *Botched,* luckily for yours truly, you'd be very wrong. I'm proud to say I just look and feel…*naturally* younger!

And that's always been my mindset: I'll do whatever I need to do, as look as I look natural. Natural is the way to be! My goal has always been to look like me…just younger. (And now my goal is to freeze my age for the next twenty years! I think I've got this!) And as I like to say: I'm in it to win it!

It's taken me a couple of decades to figure this all out, but I've learned there is nothing more helpful on the road to a fresher, more youthful version of yourself than knowing how to find the right professionals to go to and what to ask for. Well, this is your guide to all of that. Consider me your designated plastic surgery hand-holder. Together with my network of experts we can answer any and every question you've always had about needles and nips and tucks and tweaks. (Ever wonder about labiaplasty? I've had it! And did you know a lot of women actually use fillers in their outer labia to make their inner labia less prominent? I will fill you in!) Then I'm going to spend the second part of the book letting you in on all those things I do to *feel* good too. Things that will help you take care of yourself from the inside out, mentally, physically, and emotionally.

Get ready, because here we go!

HOW TO USE
THIS BOOK

Before you dive in, I want to quickly explain how to use this book to your advantage. And that's certainly not by doing every single thing that I do to look and feel young. (Unless of course you want to and are able to! When I say I've tried a lot of products, treatments, procedures, and lifestyle tactics to look and feel young... I mean *I've tried A LOT!*) Instead, I want you to use the information I've put into this book, along with my personal experiences, to help you pick and choose what things are right for *you*.

If none of them are right for you right now, financially or otherwise, that's more than okay! Even if you never want to try anything I talk about in the book, that's more than okay too! I think you'll find the topics in this guidebook to be informative regardless...and reading this book is whole lot easier than scouring through Google for hours on end to learn about these topics. (There is SO MUCH information out there on the internet and social media about this stuff and it's enough to make your head spin. Not to mention, the amount of conflicting information out there.)

It's taken me a ton of time (MANY years) and a ton of research and networking with various experts to acquire all of this knowledge and become a subject matter expert. I can definitely say, without a doubt, that it's been a full-time job! It requires a whole ton of my attention. And it's required that I do a ton of my own research to land on the right experts that I trust.

It's also cost me a lot of money, since some of the things we'll talk about can get very expensive. I realize I'm incredibly privileged to able to spend the time and the money I have, and I'm so grateful for that. I want to use all of that for good and get super honest with you about which things work and which don't, so you don't have to do it all. I know so many people who've wasted a ton of money on things that don't work—that won't be you! (For example, one of the simplest ways to cut back is by choosing affordable skincare products to use at home. Skincare does not need to be expensive to be effective—that's just a common misconception. In this book I'll give examples of lots of cost-effective options.) This book is meant to be a guide for you to hear about everything I've tried—and a few things I haven't—so you can spend your time, and hard-earned cash, wisely as well!

Life is too short to spend most of it looking old. So let me be your guide to avoid that. You can check out some of my before-and-after pictures from a few of the treatments and procedures I've tried if you flip to the middle of the book. They'll help give you a sense of the actual results you can expect if you do decide to try any of them. Go ahead and break out your highlighter and mark up this book. That's what it's here for! And again, keep in mind as you're reading that not everything we'll talk about here is right for everyone.

Follow me on Instagram @SandraLenaSilverman. I use my account to post point-of-reference videos for the different anti-aging practices I talk about in this book.

Now let's jump in and help you jump back in time!

PART ONE

LOOKING FOREVER YOUNG

CHAPTER ONE

UNLOCKING YOUR FACE'S FULL POTENTIAL

Here's the deal, ladies of certain age—and perhaps ladies who, like me, have gone through menopause or at least perimenopause: There's *no way* you're ever truly going to look like a twenty-year-old again. I know, I know, it sucks to hear that, but real life just doesn't work that way. We age, we get older, and as that earth keeps on spinning and those birthdays keep on coming, we start to look older. That's no secret, obviously, but the sooner we all accept that we'll never TRULY look twenty again, no matter *what* we do to our faces and body, no matter how much money we invest into procedures and creams, or how many jump squats we do, looking twenty is just going to be out of our reach.

In fact, let's accept it together: "We will never look twenty again!" And that is honestly okay, because if you remember, being twenty kind of sucked. Sure, you looked hot as hell, but there was too much uncertainty about life back then, too much anxiety about the future, too many boys who were terrible in bed, and, if you were like me, no money in the bank! (Girls as young as eighteen are getting Botox today, but I was raised in a middle-income family, so for me, even if Botox had existed back then, I wouldn't have been able to afford it.)

However, you know what's amazing? Being fifty. When you're fifty , things (hopefully) have pretty much come together for you. Maybe you've had a nice career, or a nice family (and you're no longer in the throes of the exhausting baby years). You have some money, you can go on nice vacations. You know what constitutes good sex, and you've proba- bly seen some sorrows, which also makes you a fully formed adult. Being fifty is fabulous! Except…for what it does to your skin. And just because you're a fully formed adult doesn't mean you don't want to look like you're thirty or forty again. That is totally attainable, and I am living proof. We may get older (and wiser of course), but we still want to look like

MILFs and vibrantly hot women. We want to rock bikinis on vacation. If we're single, we want to hook up with guys we find attractive. If we're married, we want our partners to find us attractive. And we want to have tons of energy to spend time with our friends and families, to go skiing and climb mountains and play tennis (not just pickleball!) and not feel like geriatrics. Most of all, we want to look as good as we feel, and that is an important part of this book.

Cosmetic Chronicles: Your Face, Your Beauty

How you physically look matters in this world. This is a—dare I be so cliché— *"ugly"* truth. But it's a truth, nonetheless. (I didn't make the rules, I just follow them.) And what's the very first thing people notice about how you look? Your face. And what's the very first place you start to show aging as a woman? *Say it with me now:* **Your face.** (Don't get me wrong, lots of other areas of the body are telling on a lady's age, too—chest and elbows, for instance—but your face is in the direct line of fire when people look at you.) If a woman has never been good to her skin, aging shows even faster. Think of that one girlfriend you have who's always *worshipped* the sun and has never been good about using sunblock. How does she look now, later in life? You don't even need to tell me…I can already picture it. *Like a dried-up raisin!*

When I look at the big picture, I always think of the face first and foremost. Even if you've picked up this book with zero intention of ever getting an injectable, or plastic surgery of any kind, there are lots of things you can do to keep the skin on your face looking more youthful. At bare minimum, it starts with the right skincare.

I'm alarmed every time I talk to a woman my age who doesn't have a skincare routine. A-larmed! Whether you care about looking younger or not, some things are just plain logic. If you're just lathering up any ol' bar of soap from the shower you share with your husband (that's been *everywhere* on his body… come on!) to wash your face day and night, I hope this is your wake-up call. IT'S TIME TO INVEST IN A SKINCARE ROUTINE!

Before I get all preachy, I'll let you in on a secret: I barely paid attention to my skin until my mid-twenties, let alone did I have a "skincare routine." I just washed my face with the products my mom used—whatever was lying around—and thought little else of it. I grew up in Baltimore, Maryland where I also lived my entire adult life until moving, in the fall of 2015, to Miami Beach with my husband, Dave, and two kids, Zakary and Zara (Zara is adopted from Russia, just like I was). I braved cold winters there just waiting on my beloved hot summer days where I could bake in the sun. No sunblock. Like, ever. I'd let myself literally roast out there. (The deep pigmentation on my face and chest that I now constantly fight with lasers hates me for this!)

There wasn't a specific Ah-ha! moment that knocked some sense into me, it just happened slowly in my late twenties. Before I even realized what happened, I found myself using sunblock regularly, and I never looked back. Obstacle Number 1, overcome. And it was easy.

It was probably around that same time that I started to notice a fine line here and there on my face—nothing major, but enough for me to stop picking up whatever drug store face cleanser that was on sale and step up my game. But even after committing to a skincare line, I wasn't over-the-top about using it. If I skipped some steps in the morning or at night, no biggie. I eventually defaulted yet again to the habit of just slapping on a choice moisturizer, something generic with SPF, before I headed out of the house for the day. Before bed, if I remembered, I'd also slap some night cream on and cross my fingers that I'd look tighter and brighter in the morning. Guess what? That never happened! (If this sounds like you, trust me, you're not alone. So many women I talk to are this way, and you too can be reformed!)

Now though, decades later, I'm obsessed with skincare products and am *so* consistent with my routine. You'll notice throughout this book that this is a big theme for me and should be for you too in the battle against aging—***consistency***—with skin care, treatments, supplements (I SWEAR by peptides—it's like the fountain of youth, but we'll get to that later), workouts, diets, and everything in between. I'm sure the reason the facelift I got several years ago still looks so great is because I'm very consistent with everything else I do to look young.

Over the years I've found what works best for my skin by trying an outrageous number of products (in general, I've found the best skincare products come from Korea), and also by leaning on the experts for their take. Who knows better about what products to use than an esthetician?

I've found guidance in my facialist Mindy Kim, at Mindy Kim Skincare here in Miami (www.mindykimskincare.com). She's a licensed esthetician whose been helping women like me achieve their best skin for more than ten years. I started seeing her when I first moved to Miami and let me tell you this: She is my guru. She. Is. A. Genius. You get the point! She's helped save my skin in more ways than one. Whenever I'm at her office (I typically see her every two weeks) I press her on the latest and greatest products. She's also helped me perfect my routine—precisely what I need to do every morning and night to achieve dewy skin.

Before we get into it, I'll say this: I know good skincare can be expensive…but it doesn't *have* to be! There are lots of affordable options out there. And even Mindy agrees! Sure Botox, filler, and lasers are godsends when it comes to wrinkle-free, gorgeous skin, but they're still not going to help you if your skin is flaky and pasty. So, skincare (which lotions you put on your face each day and night) is essential. Keep in mind that everyone's skin is different and will react to different products in a unique way. So finding what's best for you and your skin is all about trial and error.

Here is Mindy's expert take on what every woman (no matter the age!) should be doing to keep their skin dewy and beautiful.

SKINCARE
Words from the Wise:
Mindy Kim, Licensed Esthetician

Everyone should start being good to their skin as early as possible, and that means committing to a great skincare routine. This also means getting regular facials to exfoliate dead skin and refresh the face. I recommend finding a facialist in your area who you can trust who can tailor treatments to benefit your skin.

When a new client comes to me, we start by talking about their specific skin issues and needs. I then recommend the best treatment for them based on their skin goals, skin type, and budget. Usually, this tailored approach will include customized facials and other treatments like chemical peels, microneedling, laser treatments, or Hydra-Facials. I always make sure to explain exactly what I'm recommending and why. We take downtime into consideration, too, as certain treatments can take a few days to heal from. For example, I have some clients who are models and actresses who are often going on shoots and can't afford the downtime certain peels can have. There can be lots of shedding skin and redness.

I also educate my clients on at-home skincare. I recommend treating every morning and nighttime routine as if you're giving yourself a mini facial. Take your time applying your products and massaging them in your skin. That massaging motion contributes to collagen production, which can help tighten your skin over time. (Keep in mind that any skincare product that markets itself as a "miracle" for drastic skin tightening when used on its own is not being truthful. It takes a lot to keep your skin healthy, radiant, and tight, and one product on its own will not achieve that for you. If it sounds too good to be true, it likely is.)

Consistency is so important when it comes to a skincare routine. That's how you'll notice the biggest changes. I recommend every morning and every night using a gentle cleanser, vitamin C, a brightening serum, moisturizer, and an eye cream. And every morning, you have to apply sunblock! Particularly here in Miami where the sun can be very strong, I always educate my clients on the importance of using sunblock as part of their daily skincare routine. But using sunblock every day is a must no matter where you are. Lots of people forget to use it when they're on ski trips, for example, and they'll come off the mountain burnt.

When it comes to products for an everyday skincare routine, a lot of people think the more expensive the product, the better it is. This is not always the case. There are lots of budget-friendly options out there at your local drug store that work great. If you're on the market for new products, I recommend you try different ones and see what works best for you. Keep in mind that your skin will get used to certain products after a while, so it's important to switch them up every now and then. I recommend that you switch products once you've gone through three full bottles of a given brand. You can switch back to it in the future, of course, but give your skin a break from it and it will increase the effects.

I get asked a lot about what's new in skincare. Skincare technology is always advancing. If you find a facialist you trust in your area, they'll be able to help you determine what new treatments are best for you, and what ones are worth passing on. The exciting part is that, as the technology advances, the more customizable the treatments become.

The most important message I have is this simple reminder: Be good to your skin. Beyond your regular skincare routine and visits with a facialist you trust, be sure to treat your skin extra kindly after things like sun or weather exposure. If you've been outside in very hot or very cold conditions, take action once you're inside. Moisturize or try an at-home mask or exfoliation. This will help your skin to recover and repair, and it will prevent long-term damage.

The Skincare Sanctuary

Now that you know what Mindy recommends, let me walk you through my own skincare routine based on what I learned from her (it has ten steps, so don't be afraid to devote a little time to this process). To me, skincare is sacred. I've switched up over the years (again, it's important to do trial and error) and I've tried lots of brands on the hunt for what's best for my skin.

I recently met a woman named Amy Brodsky on a holiday trip in Cabo San Lucas, Mexico and it was like the stars aligned. Amy is a dermatologist who developed her own skincare line, Derma Made, during the pandemic. She recommended I try the products, and....They. Are. FABULOUS! I'm obsessed. Right now, I primarily use Derma Made (prices for most of the products are between $50 and $120).

Again, there are lots of skincare lines out there, so go with whatever is right for your skin and your wallet. Some affordable (yet excellent!) brands include: The INKEY List (most items are less than $20 each), COSRX (most items are less than $30 each), Seoul Ceuticals (most items are ~$20; this is an example of a great Korean skincare line), and The Ordinary (most items are less than $20). All of these can be found online with a quick Google search.

Here are the skincare routine steps I recommend with whatever products you choose:

Step 1: Cleanse

I start with Derma Made's Light Foaming Cleanser. It's imperative to clean your face every morning, even if you don't wear a ton of makeup. We sweat when we sleep, and that sweat, oil, and other debris like dust (I don't care how clean your house is, there is still dust settling on your face as you sleep!) get into your pores overnight and clog them up. So, when you scrub all that away, it means serums and other lotions have a better chance of penetrating the skin. Exfoliating cleansers get the job done. It may sound harsh for your skin, but today's exfoliators are gentle—don't scrape your skin like they did when we were younger. (Remember the one product with ground up apricot pits in it? That completely tore up my teenage skin!) Just make sure you're buying something that says "gentle."

Step 2: Hydrate

Once my skin is fully exfoliated, I spray on a hydrating mist. It's super soothing after exfoliation, and it tones the skin, calming any inflammation and providing a more even-looking complexion. Again, you don't have to use this brand, but you shouldn't skip this step. It's part of a skincare regimen for a reason; so find yourself a toner you like and stock up on some cotton balls, or do what I do—use a spray so it's quick and easy.

Step 3: Vitamin C Serum

I coat my face and neck with Derma Made's Anti-oxidant C Serum +. It's not cheap—Derma Made's is $108 for one ounce—but it packs a major punch. If you're not using a vitamin C on your skin yet, the time to start is now. It delivers a ton of antioxidant benefits. I've heard a lot of women skip this step, but Mindy tells me *absolutely not!* She said Vitamin C is important for the face, especially as we age, since it can help brighten those dreaded dark spots and promote collagen production.

Step 4: Firming Serum

It's time for serum number two. Does this seem excessive? Maybe it is to some, but it's easy to layer serums; this is a skin firming serum, which should be applied after the vitamin C. This really tones my skin, and smoothes it out. I can actually see a firmer texture and overall appearance. It also brightens the skin and evens out any redness or pigmentation problems.

Step 5: Brightening Serum

The next step is applying a brightening serum. Is it overkill to use yet another serum? Hell no! I'm living proof that you can never have too many serums at once!

Step 6: Firming Fluid

Step number six (stay with me) is firming fluid. If you want to skip this step, that's fine, but I like to add this serum on top of the others. It deeply hydrates my skin, and helps the other serums to penetrate further. Of course, it's also okay to stop applying after the first few serums.

Step 7: Moisturizing Oil

Now it's time to moisturize. I love Bio-Oil because it works amazingly well, and it's priced just right at only $14! It's so nice on the skin and gives it the best, dewiest glow—but without feeling or looking greasy like a lot of face oils. It's packed with natural oils like vitamin E to help maintain healthy looking skin and natural chamomile and lavender oil to calm and soothe. It helps combat all the dryness and leaves my skin looking soft and supple.

Step 8: Eye Cream

Now it's time for the eyes. You can use any eye serum you like but having a separate product for the eyes is important. The ingredients in eye creams are much gentler for the thin skin around your eyes. I like the Derma Made Multi-Peptide Eye Cream because it feels gentle on my delicate skin and firms it up. I dab it underneath the eyes, on the sides, and on the top of the eyelids (but with extra soft pressure). Never rub the skin around your eyes.

Step 9: Moisturize

The next step is to apply moisturizer. If it sounds crazy to go through so many steps before getting to the actual moisturizer, at least TRY this routine for a week and then see if it makes a difference. I guarantee that it does. My favorite moisturizer is the Derma Made Nia-genic Lotion. It's not outrageously expensive and it hydrates and tightens at the same time. Plus, it's a natural retinol alternative, so it's not irritating.

Step 10: Sunblock

The sun is our skin's worst enemy! And burns from our younger lives can come back and haunt us later (as mine have!). I don't care how old you are right now—even if you're a teenager reading this book— do not skip this step…ever! You can't leave this out. You've heard it your entire adult life, and it's true— you have to wear sunblock *everyday* you go outside. I personally use the EltaMD Tinted Face Sunblock with SPF 40 (only about $40) or the Derma Made SPF 50 Moisturizer Tinted (which only costs a bit more at $68). I also apply the CeraVe sunblock stick with zinc throughout the day. I take it all a step further and wear a hat or sun shielding visor when I'm outside. These Miami sun rays are strong and can prune me up! Not taking that risk.

I follow this same routine at night before I go to bed, which means I don't need to invest in specific "nighttime" formulas—and that makes things easier. (Well, as easy as a ten-step skincare routine can be!) The only additional product I use at night is Retinol—I apply a very small amount—*peasized*—to any dark spots and/or problem areas and follow this with hydroquinone, and then the final moisturizing step.

Some of these products are expensive; others are not. I pick and choose the products that work for my skin—and my budget. It's definitely not necessary to blow all of your money on skincare products. It's really about using whatever products work well for *your* skin and spending that dedicated time to massage in the products like a mini facial, as Mindy told us.

I mentioned how Amy created the Derma Made line of products using her extensive knowledge as a dermatologist, so I thought it was important to include her perspective on skincare too. Here is Amy's take on the importance of a skincare routine in our *grueling* battle against age.

SKINCARE

Words from the Wise:
Amy Brodsky, Dermatologist

Finding the right skincare routine and the right products can be challenging, since there are so many people out there telling you conflicting information. Think of how many influencers on social media alone are promoting products to you every day. A lot of products being pushed out there have ingredients that simply don't work, and the people behind those products aren't always trust-worthy. I recommend getting sound advice from a true expert, like your dermatologist or someone else you trust, like your facialist/esthetician. Think of it like this: Your skin is your largest canvas, and skincare is the paintbrush. To make sure you look the best you can, skincare is so important!

My background is in biomedical engineering, and I eventually merged my passion for science with my love for dermatology and created my own skincare line. My patients (and our customers) have found it very effective and affordable. We put our line through over 350 iterations before we perfected our final products, so we know what we're putting out there is the best it can be for our customers.

No matter your skin type and issues, I recommend a good cleanser to begin your routine every morning and night, then exfoliation at least two or three times per week. I recommend a brightening serum—ideally something with Vitamin C—followed by eye cream, moisturizer, then sunblock in the morning (and throughout the day, especially if you'll be in the sun). With this routine and our products (and some customizations depending on skin type), our customers are getting really great results within six weeks.

Beyond the products in my daily skincare routine, I also use an LED mask (I love the Omnilux Contour Face mask, specifically) for ten minutes every day—usually during my morning sessions with my personal trainer, Vanessa Reggiardo (@vanereggia_fit on Instagram), after we've worked out and done our lymphatic drainage work (which we'll detail in Chapter 11).

Oh! And if the skin on your body is in need of some extra TLC, there are a couple of things I recommend. The first is Wendala's Body Scrub ($22-$24). You can use it in the shower by working it in circular motions all over your body—it's an excellent exfoliant. The second is something I've been using lately that's very simple: olive oil. The monosaturated fatty acids and antioxidants found in olive oil have moisturizing properties that have taken my arms and legs from dry and scaly to dewy and smooth. I use a generous amount on my arms and legs once in the morning and once at night. Also, as a rule of thumb, whatever I'm putting on my face I put on my hands, including the LED light treatments. Hands are an area of our bodies that can *really* show our age if we don't take care of them.

Farewell, Chipmunk Cheeks! (And Goodbye Puffy Eyes & Jaw Too)

Besides incorporating the basics of daily skincare, another way to ease into looking your best is depuffing that face! Vanessa and I really hit strides with our lymphatic drainage protocols during the COVID-19 pandemic and it's been life changing. Basically, my lymphatic system is f*cked because of the number of surgeries I've had. Turns out, surgical procedures can sometimes mess with the lymphatic vessels and fluid won't flow in the body as it normally would. Don't get me wrong, the surgeries have been *well worth it!* But I've needed some targeted help on my body and face (and daily, at that!) to keep the fluids moving and prevent me from perpetually blowing up the size of a float in the Macy's Thanksgiving Day Parade.

The face is the worst for me. Maybe you can relate: My face swells up at even the *thought* of salt (and next up often come the hands and ankles… oh my!). There is nothing that peeves me like a bloated face. It looks so…unnatural. And it feels so…uncomfortable.

Story time! Ahead of my husband's fiftieth birthday party, I decided to get a series of those nutrition-filled IV bags. You know the ones I'm talking about? They even have entire storefronts dedicated to these kinds of places now promising to *Cure your hangover! Increase your energy! Detox the body! Enhance your immune system!*

For me, it just bloated my face so badly. I did four IVs over the course of a few days and by the day of the party, I woke up unrecognizable. My *entire face* was swollen. I looked like a freakin' bowling ball and I didn't have a clue what to do about it. Our guests kept coming up to me at the party with their expressions all crooked, asking if I was okay. *Of course I wasn't ok!* I looked hideous. I vowed to: (1) never, EVER do those IVs again… you couldn't pay me. But also (2), to figure out some solutions for face bloat so I'd never have to see that puffed-up version of me again.

I started with Gua Sha stones. If you're unfamiliar with these, I'll give you a little background. *Gua Sha* is an ancient Chinese technique for massaging the face. It's done using a smooth stone tool that's made of rose quartz or jade and it's highly effective in promoting lymphatic drainage, amping up blood circulation, and reducing inflammation. Properly using the stone—and again, being *consistent* with it—can leave your face looking *snatched!* You can buy a stone right on Amazon.

I will say, though, that Vanessa and I have broken one too many stones doing lymphatic drainage together (if they drop, they'll usually crack), so we recently switched to the FaceGym's Multi-Sculpt High-Performance Contouring Tool (worth every penny of the $69 it sells for). It's the same shape as the Gua Sha stones, but it's made of stainless steel… and unbreakable! If you're looking for a cheaper version of this FaceGym tool, just do a quick search on Amazon for "stainless steel Gua Sha" and you'll see a bunch of great options pop up there for about $10. Just make sure to read the reviews!

Here's how I use Gua Sha stones or the Face-Gym tool:

- **Start with a clean face and clean stone**: I do my entire skincare routine before using the tool in the morning. I'd also clean the stone using a mild soap and water and dry it with a cloth.

- **Master your technique:** Hold the tool at an angle to mold your face (at about 15-degrees) and gently stroke upward on the areas of the face that puff up easily. For me those were the cheekbones, jawline, and under my eyes. Repeat these strokes for about ten minutes for the best results. (Don't be shocked if you feel the burn a bit as you're doing this. I love that tingling feeling; makes me feel like something is really happening.)

- **Repeat regularly**: I do this every day. But if daily does not work for you, two to three times a week is a great place to start. Then, be…you guessed it…consistent!

For sculpting and lifting purposes, I also love FaceGym's Pure Lift Face, *The Instant Non-Invasive Facelift Tool*. It uses triple-wave technology that sends electrical impulses deep into the skin to stimulate the muscles in the face. It feels a bit strange at first, so they recommend starting at the lowest setting. I use it in upward motions on my face for about ten minutes a day. This tool is expensive ($520), but if you search "microcurrent facelift tool" on Amazon you'll see alternatives for less than $50 (again, read reviews before purchasing so you know you're getting a good one).

Another trick I've come to love (and it's *free!*) is face yoga. Face yoga is, well…exactly what it sounds like—yoga for the face. Our bodies benefit from regular exercise, why shouldn't our faces get in on the fun? Face yoga involves different stretches and poses to tone and tighten, and not only can it reduce that puff (yay!), it can also help your face look a little glow-ier and more youthful too. Best of all… it's free!

Here are some poses that work for me:

- **Cheek sculpting:** Inhale deeply and puff your cheeks with air. Transfer the air from one cheek to the other, repeating for one minute to target cheek muscles and reduce puffiness.

- **Jawline definition:** Tilt your head back and push your lower jaw forward, holding for 10 seconds. Repeat to tighten muscles along the jawline.

- **Neck and chin lift:** Tilt your head back, pucker your lips, and extend them toward the ceiling. Hold for 10 seconds for a defined jawline.

While Gua Sha stones and face yoga are excellent, what I've learned with Vanessa is that targeting the whole body will benefit the face even more. Every morning she and I spend an hour putting pressure on specific points on the body. (You don't need to devote an entire hour to this, just as much time as you can spare.) If you're a super puffy gal like me, I recommend the comprehensive approach of using all of these techniques. (We'll talk more about my routine with Vanessa in Chapter 11).

My skincare routine and debloating are only the very tip of the iceberg for me when it comes to my face. I have oh-so-many more things to teach you on the topic of the face alone, but how are you feeling so far? Are you getting excited for your new and improved look? Are you ready to take it a step further? Better now than never!

CHAPTER TWO

THE POWER OF SKIN RENEWAL & REJUVENATION

A woman I know from Miami—she's probably in her late thirties—recently started to pick my brain. Like I said, my motivation to write this book came from the overwhelming number of questions I get about achieving a youthful look, so I'm fairly used to them. But this woman's question really got me thinking.

"Your face looks younger than mine!" she said. (Insert me blushing on cue.) *"I want to follow in your footsteps. I'm not ready to go under the knife yet, but I have a budget of about $10,000 to spend right now…what should I be doing?"*

I didn't take this question lightly. I thought long and hard about it. With so many things out there to do and try, I didn't want to send her down a road of pointless treatments, or ones that didn't yield the best bang for her buck. As I marinated on my answer, I realized, surely, many other women have the same question. I know lots of people who aren't ready to take the leap into surgery yet, but they have the money and the willingness to try other means.

So what, exactly, should they do? Here's what I recommended to my very kind gal pal in Miami (of course, this assumes a good at-home skincare routine is already in play—that's the *FOUNDATION*!):

- Regular dermaplaning and microneedling (as recommended by your esthetician)
- A laser treatment like CO2, Broad Band Light (BBL) laser, or Pico
- Permanent makeup like microblading (for eyebrows) and eye and lip enhancements
- Eyelash extensions
- Botox, Dysport, or another wrinkle relaxer (I know these can be controversial, as some people think it's poison in our body, but stick with me for more on that in Chapter 4.)
- Filler/threads (whichever you prefer)
- A brightening treatment, like SKINVIVE by Juvederm

I rounded up *the* experts to help me discuss these treatments in detail in this chapter and the next, because, in my humble opinion, the list I just mentioned contains the basic necessities for looking young. In the next three chapters, we'll get into detail on all of them. These treatments have become a crucial part of my overall beauty routine and are honestly the things I swear by.

We'll start here with devices and peels. (Keep in mind that there are SO MANY treatments out there—I'd bet my bottom dollar that some new treatment is popping up as I'm typing this sentence—so I'll mostly focus on the things I've tried. But there is something out there for everyone.)

Just like with my skincare routine, I didn't take any facial treatments very seriously at first. After college, I went to work for a mortgage company, and the beauty of my schedule was that I often had free time in the afternoons. One day, to kill some time, I took a drive down the street from my office, and there it was: a day spa. I could almost hear it calling my name. *Sandy*! *Will you come try us?* And I answered that call with a resounding, YES!

Soon I had become fast friends with the woman who worked there and she taught me all the current trends in facials (like glycolic peels—they were big back then and I'd buy them from her in sets of five). I knew nothing about facial treatments before, just that they were a relaxing break from my day. Before I knew it, I was addicted (but—*GO SANDY!!*—it was an addiction I'd never need to kick). I went every other week getting one thing or another. I met my husband around this time and I wanted to look the best for him, too, aside from how good I wanted to feel for *me*. I wanted a glowing, gorgeous face, and it felt easy to attain in my twenties as a day spa regular. And just like I'd done with my skincare routine, I kept the practice up from there.

There was plenty of trial and error along the way, but I eventually figured out the treatments that gave my face the best results. I now get all these regularly. In my opinion, all woman over age forty should commit to them. Let's start with dermaplaning.

Fuzz Be Gone! Dermaplaning for Smooth Skin

Dermaplaning is a treatment that uses a surgical blade to gently scrape off the top layer of dead skin cells from the surface of your skin. It also removes any fine hairs, like that pesky peach fuzz. It's completely non-invasive which means there's zero pain involved. (In fact, I find it pretty relaxing!) It's the first on my list of must-do facial treatments (literally at the top of my list I had for my friend from earlier with the $10,000 budget). I started dermaplaning in my thirties and two decades later I still get it done once every three to four weeks. That's because it's excellent for exfoliating and exposing smoother, brighter skin underneath (and the texture of my skin is better, too). I look and feel radiant and rejuvenated after my dermaplaning treatments.

Mariana Kolev (@MiamiMarianaSkincare on Instagram) is the master of dermaplaning in Miami. She's been a licensed esthetician since 2006—and this woman knows her stuff. Here is her expert take.

DERMAPLANING
Words from the Wise:
Mariana Kolev, Licensed Esthetician

Anyone interested in dermaplaning must get the treatment done by a certified professional, meaning the person should have a valid esthetician's license. The treatment involves a surgical blade that, if handled wrongly, can risk safety and precision. If you don't already have an esthetician you trust, do your research before choosing one; make sure you find a professional who is an expert with that blade.

Now that that's out of the way: My clients love dermaplaning! There are so many benefits to this type of exfoliation, including the reduction of skin imperfections and minimizing the appearance of acne scars. It also helps prevent breakouts too, as the blade removes the follicular hairs on the face that trap the pollutants that contribute to acne. Dermaplaning also helps reduce wrinkles (including undereye wrinkles) and fine lines, and promotes a more even skin tone. It really helps bring damaged skin back to life. My clients who aren't big on chemicals especially love dermaplaning because it's completely chemical-free and a gentler exfoliation method than other options. Plus, it's completely non-invasive.

For new clients, I begin their session with a consultation where we talk about the problems they're having with their skin—whether that's dry skin, scarring, wrinkles, or anything else. We also discuss if they've had anything done to their face (like Botox, filler, lifts, other treatments) and if they have any allergies. I then put them under an amplified lamp to get a good look at their skin to see what I'm working with.

Once I determine the right treatment, we get started. The session usually lasts between thirty and sixty minutes, depending on the client, and if we plan to combine their dermaplaning with another service, like microneedling or a Hydra-Facial. I first cleanse their face. Then I use the blade to remove that outer layer of dead skin and the hairs on the face. I follow the dermaplaning by applying a series of products to their skin to moisturize it. Aftercare is simple: I ask the client to avoid makeup for the rest of the day, no sun exposure for a few days and to always use a sunblock with SPF 30. I also encourage them to use a gentle cleanser and a gentle moisturizer on their face for the first few days and to avoid any harsh products. I then recommend clients come back monthly for optimal results (our skin renews every 28 days), depending on their specific skin concerns and needs.

In Miami, I have tons of clients who are regulars at all sorts of big events, and they come to me first for what they call the "red carpet facial," aka dermaplaning. Not only does the dermaplaning session enhance the skin's appearance, but it allows makeup to be applied more smoothly, resulting in an ultra-glamorous and radiant look.

Prices for dermaplaning vary depending on geographical location and the esthetician's level of experience. In general, you can expect to pay about $100 per session. Our office offers different packages that can combine treatments, like dermaplaning and microneedling, for example.

Microneedling: A Miracle for My Fellow Glow Getters

Mariana knows best, that's what I like to say! And when I'm with her for my regular dermaplaning treatments, I let her call the shots on whether I need any add-ons. Sometimes she'll combine my dermaplaning with a HydraFacial (also completely painless). Other times, I'll combine it with a treatment called microneedling. Yes, this one hurts a bit, but it sounds more painful than it is, I swear! Sure, it's a bunch of needles jabbing into your face, but you barely feel it because they numb your face ahead of time, Microneedling is what we call *minimally invasive*. And it leaves the skin looking glowy!

Microneedling (also known as collagen induction therapy) uses a tool that looks like a pen that's tip is filled with either 12 or 36 fine needles (your esthetician would know what is best for your skin). It's placed against the skin to stimulate collagen production. When the needles touch the skin, they create "micro-injuries" that stimulate the natural healing process. This promotes the production of collagen and elastin—the building blocks of healthy, youthful skin. I personally use it to (further!) prevent wrinkles and (further!) boost my skin texture. I will warn you that if you're going into a microneedling session for the first time, don't be shocked if you leave with a blotchy face, or a few spots of dried blood. They are needles being inserted on your face, after all!

MICRONEEDLING
Words from the Wise:
Mariana Kolev, Licensed Esthetician

Just like with dermaplaning, microneedling can be done on most skin types and tones. There's a lot of customization that can go into microneedling, so I tailor the treatment to the specific needs of each client. Most often, we use microneedling for wrinkle reduction, scar reduction (like acne scars), improvement of the skin's texture and tone, and reducing enlarged pores, though we can use it for plenty of other skin issues as well. Beyond the face, I also have clients who love microneedling for their neck, chest, and hands to fight aging.

Because this procedure is minimally invasive, in the days leading up to it, I recommend my clients avoid sun exposure, retinoids, and any harsh skincare products to help reduce the risk of complications. When they get to me for their session, we discuss their needs and assess their skin (I'll examine it under my amplified light, just like I do before my dermaplaning sessions). Then I begin with a numbing cream to minimize any discomfort. I let that sit for about twenty minutes, so their skin is nice and numb before we start. The microneedling itself usually lasts about thirty minutes depending on the size of the treatment area and the specific concerns we're addressing (for instance, deeper scars will take longer to work with).

Afterward, I ask my clients to avoid sun exposure for a few days, and always apply sunblock with SPF 30 (I can never stress this enough!), use a mild cleanser when washing the face, and stay hydrated. They should also avoid retinoids after treatment, until the skin has fully recovered. Costs for a microneedling session can range from $200 to $700, depending on location and experience of the esthetician. Some patients require multiple sessions to get the best results.

If you're not ready for professional microneedling, or want a cheaper option, there are some decent microneedling rollers you can purchase and use at home. (Keep in mind that the results you'll see from the at-home rollers will be less noticeable than the ones you'd get from professional microneedling, but it's still a good alternative. The at-home ones are painless, too, which is another benefit.) I like the GloPRO At-Home Microneedling Tool by BeautyBio. It sells for $199 but you get at least twenty-four uses out of it (they say to use it at least three times a week and it lasts two to three months before the needles dull and it needs to be replaced). They recommend you use it on clean skin and use horizontal, vertical, and diagonal motions on all target areas of the face for sixty seconds. Then follow with a serum or moisturizer. (And again, I beg you…be cautious in the sun!)

If you're on the hunt for a cheaper version of the GloPRO tool, there are other comparable tools on Amazon in the $20 to $30 range. Again, just be sure to read the reviews so you're not purchasing one that's going to do more harm than good on your skin. Beyond the face, I like to use my at-home microneedling tool on my knees; it helps keep that skin looking rejuvenated.

Peeling Back Those Years

When it comes to facial peels, I've tried them all. My favorites are the retinol peel and the chemical peel that my facialist Mindy Kim offers at her office in the Miami area. I recommend researching to find your own Mindy Kim wherever you are. (Like I've said, she's a critical part of my anti-aging routine!) Of course, you want the treatments to be done the best they can be, but you also want to find someone who is going to do them well (meaning someone who isn't a scam artist). I've been down some major rabbit holes with specialists who looked good on the surface but would do things to my face and body that made me look *worse*, just so I'd come back and spend more with them. I've even gotten referrals from friends who've turned out to be absolute disasters. Nothing is as important as this: DO. YOUR. RESEARCH.

If you're in my area, you cannot go wrong with Mindy. Here is her explanation of a couple of different peels she does at her office.

POPULAR PEELS
Words from the Wise:
Mindy Kim, Licensed Esthetician

A popular peel I offer to help fight aging is a retinol peel. (Note: These require expertise from a trained, certified professional.) During the consultation, we tailor the retinol concentration and treatment plan. On average, depending on where you are in the country, a single retinol peel session can range from $100 to $300. I personally charge $300 for an hour-long retinol peel.

Another option my clients like is a more generalized chemical peel. This peel contains various acids like glycolic or salicylic acid. Similarly, they begin with a consultation where we talk about the skin's needs and customize the chemical peel to address specific concerns. I also do extractions during the chemical peel. Generally, prices range from $100 to $300 per session. I currently charge $255 for an hour.

Another type of peel I've tried is the VI peel (short for Vitality Institute Peel) which is intended to help with skin's texture and tone. The peel has a mix of ingredients, including TCA (Trichloroacetic Acid), Retin-A, salicylic acid, phenol, and Vitamin C, that work together to exfoliate the skin. It also helps to stimulate collagen production and fight fine lines and wrinkles, acne, and sun damage. It can be used on any skin type. The VI peel burns a little but isn't overly painful. On average, it costs between $200 and $500 per treatment and they take anywhere from twenty to forty-five minutes. They're safe to get every four to six weeks. Truthfully, lots of people love the VI peel but I did not like it for my face. I'll still use this type of peel for other parts of my body, but doubt I'll do it on my face ever again. To each their own! But something worth looking into.

As for an at-home peel, I love the Jessner's Chemical Peel, which you can find online for as little as $12. I use it once every two weeks. A warning for those who want to try it—it does make your skin peel. It exfoliates the top layer of the skin to enhance skin texture and tone, so you'll definitely notice that top layer coming off. Do not, and I repeat, *do not* go out in the sun for a few days after you use it. Use the same caution with the sun that you'd use if you'd gotten a professional peel.

Another peel I love to use at home is the 70% Glycolic At Home Adjustable Peel which sells for only $15.99. (Just do a quick Google search and you'll be able to find it.) It's great for lighter skin tones like mine and can be used wherever on the body. For darker skin tones, the brand recommends their 30% Glycolic acid mixture. No matter which one you're using, be sure to follow the directions carefully for the best results.

Lasers Are for You

I love everything about looking young, but there's one treatment I may love above all else for my face, and that's lasers. Let's start with the CO2 laser (this is for lighter skin tones and isn't recommend on darker skin. For darker skin tones, the Pico laser is an excellent alternative, which we'll get to shortly). Put simply, the CO2 laser uses light to remove deeper layers of the skin, well beyond what's possible with dermaplaning or other treatments. The laser can be aggressive—it's used directly against your skin and feels like a burn. There are customizations, and even a "light" setting, but either way it hurts…I won't lie to you. But the results are really great for scarring, overall complexion, improved texture, tightening, and things like smokers' lines and other deep lines. When it heals, your skin is silky-smooth. (Honestly, I haven't had the best results with the CO2 laser for pigmentation, though. I'll talk about the laser I like best for pigmentation—the Broad Band Light (BBL) laser—shortly.)

One of the top uses for the CO2 laser is acne scarring (and it can remove other scars on your body, too—more on this later in the book). I've used this laser treatment to prevent aging on my chest and have had good results.

I got my first CO2 laser treatment in my early forties back in Baltimore, but it wasn't very aggressive, so I didn't notice much of a change in my skin. In Miami, I go to the best of the best— Amy Koberling, a dermatology physician assistant at Baumann Cosmetic Dermatology (she's @amykoberling on Instagram and she also has a podcast on all things skincare called *#skinthusiast: the podcast*). Amy's results are freaking amazing. Here's her take on the CO2 laser:

CO2 LASER

Words from the Wise:
Amy Koberling,
Dermatology Physician's Assistant

The CO2 laser offers two very different treatment options: the light laser and the deeper fusion laser. Both treatments are very customizable. Given how customizable the CO2 laser is, there's no real age range for an "ideal candidate." For instance, I've treated women in their eighties with the CO2 laser on deep fusion mode to really tighten the skin and help with wrinkles. But I've also had a patient in her early thirties who I treated with the laser on light mode. So, it depends on the state of the skin, the goals of the patient and their skin concerns, and our professional take as well.

Patients who want the deeper fusion laser are usually ones I've been seeing at our office for some time. We've thoroughly discussed their interest in CO2, and their concerns—like sagging skin, texture, fine lines, wrinkles, or anything else. Sometimes they're interested in more collagen production and the laser can help with that too. Maybe they have signs of photoaging—like brown spots.

No matter what, I discuss everything with them thoroughly, so they know what they're getting into. Then I discuss with the patient how motivated they are because this laser can be a little intense. There is downtime, but the results will be a lot better than some of the other procedures we offer where the downtime is less.

I always evaluate their skin as well. Our office has a VISIA skin analysis camera and I use that to look at their skin closely; it shows me things that can't be seen with the naked eye such as the level of sun damage and the deeper level of redness in the skin. The VISIA also gives a "wrinkle score," which basically compares that client's skin to that of people across the country and spits out a percentile, say their skin is 90 percent better in wrinkles than others their age, or in some cases, 20 percent better. This all helps me determine the best treatment.

We also tailor the treatment for different areas of the face. Around the mouth where people are more likely to have those fine "smokers' lines," we can be a bit more aggressive with the laser compared to the rest of the face. It's really all about customizing the treatment for the patient. I've never performed the same CO2 treatment on two patients—it's all customized.

Once we decide on a treatment, I prepare the patient as much as possible by showing them a lot of before-and-after pictures so they know what to expect. (If you've ever seen what a patient's skin looks like directly after the treatment, it can be alarming. But after a couple weeks of healing, the skin looks amazing.) It looks scarier than it feels, but I want my patients to be fully prepared.

I'm very passionate about topical skin care, so every patient starts with a topical regimen. But if there's a new client I've done a consultation with and they decide they're going to do the CO2 laser, I ensure that they're following a solid skin care routine leading up to the procedure. This includes Vitamin C, sunblock, and retinoids. (I'll then ask them to stop the retinoids a few days before the CO2 laser procedure is scheduled.)

Also, if somebody is prone to hyperpigmentation, I want them on some sort of pre-treatment that's going to calm down those pigment-making cells, so we don't end up with a flare-up after the laser. All of this helps increase our potential results. We don't want immediate sun exposure before any sort of laser, especially if the patient is prone to hyperpigmentation, because that means those pigment-making cells are activated and on alert. Then, if you injure the skin, they're much more likely to hyper-pigment.

If a patient comes to me who simply can't stay away from the sun, I will rarely do a procedure like this on them for a couple of reasons. First, I need to be able to trust that they're going to be fully out of the sun while they're healing because of the potential complications. Second, if they're not committed to less sun or no sun exposure, there's really no point in wasting their money on this laser because all the issues are going to come back. If this person was a sun worshipper previously, but is now ready to change, I'll do it. But if it's someone who is going to go right back in the sun after they heal, then it's not the right treatment for them. I will say, most of the patients who see me are super motivated when it comes to their skin care, so it's rare that I have to lecture a patient about sun exposure. They're usually on top of it already.

Some patients are nervous when they come in for their first CO2 laser procedure. For the pain, we apply a strong numbing cream and then let the patient sit with it on their face for about twenty to thirty minutes to let their face numb. Then, depending on the patient, I might offer some sort of oral medication or even an oral anxiolytic to help them, which we'll administer while they're at the clinic. We also have a pronox machine, which is nitrous oxide or laughing gas similar to what you'd get at the dentist. We use a combination of the cream, oral medication, and pronox, as appropriate for the specific patient. Pain tolerance varies for each patient. Some patients do the treatment without issue, while others are rather uncomfortable. The majority of patients feel pretty good and are able to tolerate the treatment without any breaks, while others who experience a lot of pain will request a break midway through.

The procedure takes between thirty minutes and a couple of hours, depending on the customized treatment we've developed. These are fractional lasers, meaning that microscopic areas of the skin are treated, and then other microscopic areas are left untreated. We tailor that ratio based on the person. By only treating the right microscopic areas for them, this allows the healthy skin cells from the surrounding areas to come in. That's what's impactful when it comes to decreasing the healing time and the risk of complications with some of the more intense lasers.

I will say that, for my first-timers, they often have a What did I do? moment when they see their face immediately after the procedure (it will look severely sunburned). But the final results are so amazing that once they heal, they always come back.

If the patient wants optimal results, then aftercare should be taken seriously, especially when it comes to limiting sun exposure. We give our patients detailed instructions to follow when they leave: For the first few days, the only thing that should be used on the skin is Aquafor or Vaseline to keep the skin moist. After that, we give them a simple regimen to follow which is a very gentle cleanser and a very gentle moisturizer. They can still use Aquafor, and if they'll be in the sun at all for whatever reason, a form of physical sunblock to cover their face. I tell my patients that, for the first few days, I'd rather they be indoors with their blinds closed—stay out of the sun. If they get sun exposure, the complications can be worse.

A lot of times my patients will take time off work, especially if they are private and don't want people to see the scabbing that results as the skins begins to heal. Other patients don't mind as much and are more tolerant of being out in public. We recommend two full weeks before patients resume their regular skincare regimen. Once they do, I make sure they're using retinoids as part of their routine, as these further compound the collagen production that began in the skin after the laser.

How often patients repeat the laser treatments depends on several factors, such as specific skin concerns, the age of the patient, and how aggressive a treatment we did. If the treatment was aggressive, I like to space treatments out with a couple of years in between, but of course that depends on the patient. If there's somebody with severe or significant laxity, or lots of fine lines and wrinkles, this laser is something they're going to want to do more often, perhaps multiple times a year once the skin is fully healed. I personally do it about once a year at the most.

I'll end on this final thought: It's very, very important to have a professional do this. It cannot be done otherwise, under no circumstances!

So, the CO2 laser can be a pain, but it's worth it, and not just for my face and chest! I've recently done CO2 on some scars I have on my elbows from an elbow lift procedure (we'll get to that procedure), and it's helped a lot so far. Amy recommended between four and five sessions for the elbow scars. As far as cost goes with the CO2 laser, it usually ranges between $2,000 and $5,000 per session on the face, with the lighter laser treatments costing on the lower end. Elbows cost about $700 per session.

Now what if you have darker skin and want something similar for your face? The **Pico laser** is a great option for that. One of my closest friends, Susan Ra (she's a cosmetic dentist you'll hear from in the next chapter) has darker skin, and gets Pico. She really likes it. I talked to her about her experience, and she told me she goes about once a year and has great results from it. Similar to CO2, they'll use a numbing cream on her skin beforehand for the pain.

How does Pico work? The Pico laser produces short pulses of light onto the skin to rejuvenate it and help treat pigmentation (like dark spots), and other skin issues. The laser breaks the pigment down, helping the body to naturally eliminate it. I've gotten this laser for a few stubborn sunspots on my face and it's worked pretty well. I've done it a couple of times so far and the spots are significantly less noticeable. Because it's been focused on specific spots for me rather than the entire face, the pain is far less than the CO2 laser. Amy numbs the spots she is going to laser, and we zap! Prices for the Pico laser vary a lot: They can be as low as $300 a session and up to about $1,500 a session. Most people need multiple sessions to get the results they want.

Remember I mentioned how I kicked myself because of the sun exposure I got in my early twenties? I've turned to the **Broad Band Light (BBL) laser** to fight that damn pigmentation for good! I had a sunspot on the side of my face for *years* that would not go away. I started to fixate on it to the point where I couldn't see anything else when I looked in the mirror. Plus, NOTHING worked (I tried it all, as you can imagine!). Then Denise Santoli, another of my trusted experts based here in Miami (www.floridacentercosmetic.com), suggested we try the BBL laser.

The BBL laser works similarly to the Pico laser, but there's a specific setting on the machine for sunspots and pigmentation. Well…it worked! And it did its job after only one session. At first the spot she blasted looked like sprinkled pepper on my face, but after a few days, it all disappeared. I'll continue to use this for any pigmentation issues for sure. (It's very painful, but I didn't use a numbing cream for this, so that could be why. I'd recommend asking for numbing, especially if you're going to use it for a larger area.) My assistant also tried the BBL laser for both pigmentation and rosacea, and had great results with it too. If you have rosacea, it's definitely worth looking into!

The **Halo laser** is popular too. I haven't personally tried it, but I definitely would. As with other lasers, the Halo laser can help with wrinkles and fine lines, acne and other scars, and sun damage. There's less downtime with the Halo compared to the CO2. The treatment usually takes between thirty and sixty minutes (and, of course, the skin is numbed beforehand) and the downtime is usually only about three to five days. Results are usually seen within a week.

IPL (Intense Pulsed Light) is another common treatment to fight pigmentation, though not technically a laser. It's a light-based treatment where the light is absorbed by the tissues it's targeted on. This causes heat there that—in addition to fighting pigmentation—can stimulate collagen production, reduce hair growth (so it's often used for hair removal in places on the body) and it can even treat spider veins. I've never personally tried this, though I would for sure (remember, I'll try *anything!*)

Now, lasers are wonderful, but I will make a couple of important points. First, you *must* be careful with the sun after laser treatments, and I'm not just talking about directly after the procedure—I mean long term. There's no point in spending the money and time, and experiencing the pain, to do these if you're going to ruin the effects with sun exposure. For example, even several minutes of direct sun on the small spot where I used BBL can bring that pigmentation all back. Beyond sunblock, I bought a UV protection sun shielding visor hat that I wear anytime I'll be in the sun. You can find them on Amazon for less than $30. They look ridiculous—when you see one, you'll know what I mean—but you'd rather look silly in this visor than have your skin look crappy!

And second, using professional lasers can too often make your skin very thin. Think about it… you're essentially burning off layers, so doing too many treatments spaced too closely together will make your skin look almost, well, *translucent.* Eek!! I've seen women who've done this, and honestly it gives me goosebumps even thinking about it. Please, please, *please* consult with a trusted and vetted expert on how often to wait between treatments if you plan on doing these lasers. (I've heard that when used too often, Ultherapy—an alternative to lasers that uses ultrasounds therapy to tighten skin—tends to leave the skin extra thin, especially when used on the neck. I've never done it and don't plan to for that very reason. I never want to do anything that would make my skin difficult to work with when I go for a facelift re-up down the road!)

Now what about at-home lasers? Do they exist? Excitingly, YES! I told you in Chapter 1 that I use the Omnilux LED mask ten minutes a day, every day, and it's helped my skin so much.

Another laser that's popular for at-home use is the Medicube AGE-R Booster Pro 6-in-1 skin care booster (it sells for $384). It has several different LED light color options depending on your skin goals. It has the red light treatment for skin tightening and skin elasticity, and it also has these light color options for these purposes:

- Blue: Pore care & sebum control
- Orange: Brightening
- Green: Volumizing
- Purple: Boosts skincare

Medicube also sells a giftbox that includes that laser along with their AGE-R Glutathione Glow Serum which they recommend using with it. In my opinion, it's definitely worth exploring if you're interested.

I haven't tried it, but I've been hearing a lot lately about a really powerful at-home laser called the LYMA laser. It's a tool that, like other lasers, helps with fine lines and other signs of aging (you can even use it around the delicate skin around your eyes; no goggles needed). It's FDA-approved and it's said to be one hundred times more powerful than LED light. The LYMA laser looks like a little wand, and you swipe it over your skin, repeating the movement five times over each area, and you can use it every day on any aging areas of your body. I've seen before-and-afters of people's jowls, for instance, and oh my God! Remarkable! Another huge benefit is that it's completely painless—it actually feels cold instead of giving off tons of scorching hot heat. It's expensive, selling for $2,695 at the time I'm writing this, but when you think of how much use you can get out of it, it seems worth it. (Note that, although far stronger than an LED light, this laser won't make your skin thin the same way professional lasers would, so there's no harm in everyday use.) It gets really good reviews, so if you're not ready to invest in the professional lasers just yet, this is a great alternative.

All of these are helpful options! With so many day spas out there promising all kinds of treatments to leave you looking younger, the devices, peels, and lasers I discussed here are really the ones to trust.

CHAPTER THREE

MILLION DOLLAR SMILE & PERMANENT MAKEUP

How else can we improve the face in a minimally invasive way? Well, I'm happy you asked! I've got a few other tricks up my sleeve for you before we even get to injectables (which is a topic I feel passionate about—I'm sure you figured as much).

Let's start with those teeth! Something I didn't include in my list of "must dos" for a $10,000 budget is dentistry. This is because, well, cosmetic dentistry costs *A LOT* of money. But I still think it's worth talking about, because a smile can tell a *major* tale when it comes to overall beauty.

A Good Smile Speaks Volumes

Some women were simply born with perfection, and for me, it was my teeth. They were perfect. *P-E-R-F-E-C-T!* I knew I shouldn't mess with them, but being who I am, I couldn't help myself. After my pregnancy with my son Zakary, I noticed my bottom teeth had shifted. Every time I looked in the mirror, it was the first thing I noticed, so I went to an orthodontist in Baltimore who told me I needed braces on both the bottom *and* the top…

Why I listened to this scam artist is beyond me. But I did. And it completely threw off my bite. What's worse: My teeth started chipping now that my bite was off. It was a disaster. I was freaking out—I couldn't stop thinking about how much I missed how my old teeth looked. CURSE THOSE BRACES!!

I eventually decided it was time for veneers. Veneers are like custom-made shells for your teeth typically made of porcelain or composite resin. Dentists attach them to the front surface of your teeth to improve their shape, size, color, or overall appearance. I ended up getting eight of them, but because my bite was still off, they all started to chip and crack too.

Now I was *infuriated!* In between all of this, I had put myself through one of the worst pains of my life with gum restoration surgery. The periodontist had taken flesh from the roof of my mouth to perform the surgery. Nothing has ever hurt like that! Overall, this attempted journey back to good teeth turned out to be a failure. Crash and burn.

That's when I went to my close friend and cosmetic dentist Dr. Susan Ra, who works at Touch of Smiles Dental Care in Cockeysville, Maryland. Dr. Ra and I have been friends since college, so aside from her being highly knowledgeable and *top of class* in cosmetic dentistry, I trust her more than I trust most people in this world. She redid my veneers for me to get things looking good and fixed my bite so the tooth chipping would stop once and for all.

When I got to Miami, I was still dreaming of my old teeth. I'd look at old pictures of myself and ask, *"Why?! Why those damned braces??"* I couldn't get over it—I was a woman obsessed. Then, I found Dr. Tal Morr, a prosthodontist (a specialist in the replacement and reconstruction of teeth) and he once again had to fix my bite. But this is when the best thing ever happened…Dr. Morr worked with an artist who was able to recreate my original teeth as veneers. It was my dream come true (I paid about three times more per tooth than traditional veneers, but it was *so worth it!*). Dr. Morr also restored my gums in a couple of other areas (turns out my bite being off caused my gums to recede), but this time it was far less painful. Instead of using flesh from the roof of my mouth, he used tissue from a cadaver (don't worry, the tissue is *very* carefully processed and preserved, so it's safe). The cadaver tissues served as a graft to help my own gums regenerate. It was expensive, but like other things I've had done, *so worth it!* (Many dentists will except insurance for gum restoration, though, so if it's something you're interested in, definitely do your research.)

Not to sound like some corny advertisement, but now I smile in the mirror every chance I get. I visit Dr. Morr once every three months for a checkup, and I'm (hopefully!) set for life. And when I'm in Baltimore, I'm always sure to swing by Dr. Ra's too. If you've considered getting anything cosmetic done to your teeth, here is some of her expert insight (including an explanation of the *golden ratio* which is fascinating).

COSMETIC DENTISTRY
Words from the Wise:
Susan Ra, DDS

A lot of people don't know what they want when it comes to cosmetic dentistry. They might come into our office with an example of a look they like—a celebrity or something along those lines—or they'll tell me what about their smile they don't like. I regularly hear, "I want a full smile!" meaning when they smile, they want to see a certain number of teeth—all the premolars and incisors, maybe the beginning of a molar. I usually tell my patients what I think they need to have done. And they trust me, which is great! I also attempt to help them achieve "the golden ratio."

At a minimum, most people want their teeth whitened. When I first got out of dental school, everyone was all about the natural look for teeth. But the natural look was just…yellow. I would not want that! Eventually everyone started to catch on that white teeth look much nicer and cleaner. So, I'm happy to report that white teeth are here to stay. One of the biggest mistakes I see are people who believe they'll completely change their smile only by whitening their teeth. Changing a smile is a lot more than that. Correcting the shape is really important too.

The golden ratio is something aesthetic to the eye, meaning it makes sense to the eye. If your cheek is shaped a certain way, according to the golden ratio, your smile should follow your face that same way. When someone has the golden ratio, their smile makes sense to the eye and follows along the contours of the face. Think of certain celebrities who have perfect symmetry, like Kate Beckinsale: She has the golden ratio. Faces like that are therefore more appealing to the eye than others. When someone doesn't have it, people will see you and think your smile is off. So, when someone doesn't have the golden ratio, it means it's not pleasing to the eye (the eye can pick up on discrepancies).

More specifically, there is an ideal proportion between the visible width of the two front teeth and the width of the central incisors and lateral incisors combined. According to this idea, the width of the two front teeth should be in a specific relationship with the combined width of the adjacent teeth. In a smile that adheres to the golden ratio, the width of the central incisor (front tooth) is ideally 1.618 times wider than the width of one of the lateral incisors (the teeth next to the central incisors).

Every dentist learns about the golden ratio in dental school, but whether they put it into practice is the difference. The first thing to look for when seeking a dentist to help achieve the golden ratio is that they are someone who advertises their practice as cosmetic dentistry. Check their years of experience as a dentist, as well. Sometimes a newer dentist simply won't know what to look for yet. For example, they may put on veneers and think they look nice—truthfully, though, any veneer will look nicer than the original teeth---but they might not know to check that the veneers aren't negatively impacting the patient's speech. They also might not know to check for what's known as the curve of Spee. If the patient looks straight ahead, are their teeth parallel to the horizon, or do they go up a little bit? According to the curve of Spee, their teeth should go up a little bit on the sides, giving an uprise in the smile. When people don't have the curve of Spee, it almost looks as if their teeth are too long when they're not.

The face offers the most telltale signs of aging in women, especially for those who grind their teeth. If you're a teeth grinder, as you get older your face will sag as your teeth grind down. For these women, we raise the bite so that the corners of the mouth aren't squished (and this makes their lips look fuller, too). We'll crown all the teeth in the back to restore the height they lost.

Cosmetic dentistry can be very costly, and many people have budget issues, so in that case, we only suggest doing veneers for the top teeth. This helps give the patient a fuller smile. We'll also give them a night guard, so they don't grind their teeth. (I do not ever recommend using over-the-counter nightguards. They don't work.)

Then there is something called "snap-on smile," which is probably the worst thing I hear requests for. It's essentially a snap-on teeth cover that hides any obvious tooth decay. Often people who are out in the public with notoriety of some kind (but can't afford the real deal) request them. I don't recommend it. Another mistake I see are veneers that are too big for the person's tongue; this makes it difficult for them to speak well. If you've met someone with veneers who speaks with a lisp, you know what I mean. The right cosmetic dentist will make sure the tooth size is precise enough that the patient can pronounce certain sounds without interference.

The cost of cosmetic dental work can be high—upward of $30,000 for a full set of veneers.

There are a lot of people who don't need anything, so I'm very honest with them about that. Ultimately, my best advice to any and every person who will listen is this: Do everything you can to protect your teeth. How do you best protect them? I always advise my patients against sugary sodas and hard foods, like hard candies and pretzels, ice chewing, and nuts. (A trick I recommend for almond lovers is putting the almonds in water and then draining them and eating them soft.) Likewise, chewy candies can pull off fillings and crowns. Chewing gum will exasperate any kind of grinding and TMJ issues, and it makes those muscles in your jaw—the masseters—big too. It is, of course, also important to be diligent about brushing and flossing, and to have regular visits to your dentist.

Perfecting Those Brows with Microblading & Hybrid

Permanent makeup is another tool in my arsenal of beauty procedures. Listen, I'll get real here, it's hard for me to find the motivation to do my own makeup every day. Consider how much time I'm already spending on my face with skincare and treatments alone…I don't always have even more time left to line my brows, lip, and eyes on top of everything else. I try to make the makeup part as easy as I can on myself.

So, my eyebrows…they're microbladed. All I need to do is go over them quickly in the morning with the eyebrow pencil and I'm done. Microblading is like a semipermanent tattoo for your eyebrows that creates a fuller and more defined look. During the procedure, a trained technician uses a handheld tool with tiny needles to deposit pigment into the layers of your skin where your eyebrows are, mimicking the appearance of individual hair strokes.

I'd gotten my eyebrows tattooed in that *old school way* back in Baltimore years ago but didn't like the way it looked. Thankfully those disappeared over time. Then when I got to Miami, I found Johanna Hedman, owner and founder of The Hedman Method (www.hedmanmethod.com), and she's made me *obsessed* with my eyebrows. She and I do a hybrid of microblading and shading on mine, which she goes over in her "Words from the Wise" comments too. If you get your eyebrows microbladed in the Miami area, chances are you know (or at least know of) Johanna.

MICROBLADING
Words from the Wise:
Johanna Hedman, Board Certified
Microblading Technician

I started in the field about a decade ago. I was passionate about eyebrows because I never had any. I'm fair complexioned with very little brow and I always wondered if there was a solution for this. I didn't want to have to do my eyebrows every morning, but I would because I didn't like anybody to see me before makeup. I wanted a way to feel more confident. My husband is from Brazil and when I was there with him, I realized they were light-years ahead of where we were in the U.S. when it came to technology for the brows. I knew I wanted to get into it professionally, and that I'd be good at it too. In the U.S., everything was old-school tattooing, and there was no training or anything like that. There was an association, but the styles they taught were older techniques. So, I went to school for microblading in Brazil and got certified there.

Then I brought the techniques to the U.S. with me. I started developing a way of doing microblading that looked more natural, and, over time, I improved the process and technique. That's how I created my business, The Hedman Method, where the natural look is our signature. While we will accommodate heavier looks as requested, I would personally like to leave the brow two to three percent underdone than have something overdone. It's the Hedman way!

Anyone is an ideal client for microblading (though we don't do microblading on women who are pregnant, as a precaution). There is so much misinformation out there now about microblading. For example, a lot of people say you cannot do microblading on someone who is older. That's not necessarily true. It depends on how it's done.

If it's done very delicately and carefully, we can still have great results on older women—even women in their nineties. It's a matter of doing it the correct way and working very conservatively. We have had very good results across the board with different ages and skin types.

I have clients who have no eyebrows and I have clients who have some hair there already—either way, microblading gives them a full and shapely look. Even people with good eyebrows often want them to be the best they can. If a person has a very flattering shape, we can make the shape even better, putting an emphasis on the arch for a little bit of a lift for the eye, or manipulating the shape to fit the rest of their features. When a new client comes for their appointment, we begin with a consultation. We discuss their desired outcome and look at the features they have, their skin type, the type of hair and color. We get very clear on their objectives and then we sketch the shape so the client can see the shape and color before we start. Once they've approved it, then we go to the actual microblading. We use two kinds of numbing: One is put on the client beforehand, usually about thirty minutes before we start while they're filling out their forms. Once we've started the procedure, because the skin is a little bit open at that point, we can put on a different kind of numbing for patients who are more sensitive and who might experience pain. Most clients experience very little pain with the numbing.

While this is called microblading, the tool is not an actual blade, but a number of needles in the shape of the blade. We dip the tool into pigment to trap the pigment in between the needles, and this is etched on the skin. That's how the pigment is inserted. We deposit pigment into the skin in a way that gives the illusion of fuller eyebrows. It looks like little hairs, but that's the pigment put into the skin. Once it heals, it looks like full eyebrows.

The amount of time it takes to complete microblading depends on the specific artist. I've personally done over ten thousand procedures (and we've done over fifteen thousand in our office), so I've gotten very skilled at it and can do it fast—about two hours on average. Newer artists will take longer.

The most important rule is to go to someone who has a lot of experience. With microblading, there are a wide range of artists out there—some are very good and some not so good. When looking for a microblading artist, I recommend reading online reviews, not just what the reviews say, but the quantity of reviews (look for someone with hundreds of good reviews, instead of just twenty or thirty). Make sure whoever you go to is a board-certified artist through the American Association of Micro Pigmentation and the Society of Permanent Cosmetic Professionals.

Doing your due diligence is important to ensure your results are aesthetically pleasing, but there are other things that can go wrong if working with somebody who is not well trained or does not follow the proper hygiene to avoid cross contamination. (Because microblading involves opening the skin, there's usually a little bit of blood.) You should only patronize a place that is very careful with hygiene. Results you can sometimes fix. But who cares if you have beautiful eyebrows if you contract hepatitis? For me, safety is the most important thing. Don't be afraid to call around and interview different artists to see who you feel comfortable with. They could be an amazing artist, but if you don't feel comfortable with them, you're not going to want them doing this on your face.

For aftercare, clean the eyebrows once or twice daily with a very milky soap and then put an ointment on a few times a day. Many places will tell clients not to drink water or exercise afterward, but aftercare does not have to be that strict. We allow clients to lightly exercise that first week after treatment.

About a month later, we'll have the client return for a touchup at which point we'll reinforce everything said previously. If the client wants to make any changes to the shape or color, we can usually do that in the touch up. The touchup appointment is important in that it makes that microblading last longer. After that, another touchup won't be needed for about a year or so. The more natural results will need to be touched up more frequently, but if you go to someone who has a heavy hand—and who creates a heavy brow—those results will usually last longer. It's a tradeoff, but I recommend the natural look versus the tattooed look.

Hybrid is another popular technique for eyebrows. It's an even more natural look than the traditional microblading, and it involves both hair strokes and what's known as shading. What's good about that is that if the client doesn't have a lot of hair, or if they have a big chunk of hair, you can blend seamlessly with the hybrid technique. In those cases, with only microblading, you're going to see the areas that don't have any hair and they're going to look a little bit less natural than areas that do. Hybrid helps bridge that gap and makes it look soft and nice.

It's also something my clients choose when they want a little bit more of a dramatic brow or a little more body to the brow. They tend to like hybrid for this because we can achieve that bold and defined look while also looking natural. People come to us saying how a friend had microblading, but it doesn't look natural; they want our results because they're airier and softer looking. And it's true. Microblading can look very different if the artist is doing the hair stroke too close; it will result in looking too solid, and it no longer looks like microblading.

The cost of microblading ranges widely, and it is more expensive in bigger cities, but I would say it costs at least $700 and up. If you're looking to go to someone for less than that, it's most likely not someone who is very trained. We charge between $1,100 and $1,700, but there are places that charge up to $3,000. You might be tempted to walk into that place around the corner because they're having a $400 microblading deal. Remember, any good artist—most of the time—is going to charge what they are worth. A lot of people think microblading shouldn't be that expensive, but you're paying a highly skilled person to put something on your face.

You also want to make sure that the style of the artist has appeal to you because every artist works slightly differently. If you want a very natural look, look for somebody who works very naturally. If you want a little bit more of the bold look, look for someone whose results on clients looks bold. Check out their before-and-afters and be sure to look at the before pictures that look most like your current eyebrows so you can best understand the type of results you would get.

Microblading can be removed and there are a couple different options. One option is lasers, and the other option is saline removal. With the laser removal, there is a little more downtime and it's more intense. The laser option can also change the pigment of the skin, and sometimes it's very difficult to redo the eyebrows after laser because of the thinning affect it has on the skin. The saline option is usually a gradual process, so it takes a little longer to lift the pigment than with the laser, but the downtime is less and it doesn't affect the skin or change the texture as much.

A quick mention here that if you're someone who is looking for some extra growth of your natural eyebrows, I have friends who have used and loved RevitaBrow Advanced ($60). You apply it once a day to clean, dry eyebrows in several short strokes. People say it works within just several weeks.

Fifty Shades of Blushing

Lip blushing is something else I do with Johanna, and I love it. It's a form of permanent makeup where pigment (in this case, a color you'd want to see on your lips every day) is applied to the lips. It's like lipstick that's there all the time, without any effort on your part at all. The color enhances the lips all around and it also creates a fuller and more defined look. Eye shading does the same thing, but to your eyelids, and an eye enhancement is semi-permanent eyeliner.

All of these are equally as invasive as microblading—again, it's like tattooing. I wouldn't call it fun or relaxing, but with the numbing cream, it's not terrible. And the results last a year (and sometimes up to three years). I've personally done the lip shading and love it. For the most part during the day, I keep things very simple—just my tinted sunblock and a bit of lip gloss, and I'm set for the day. With permanent makeup, you really don't have to wear much.

LIP BLUSHING, EYE SHADING & EYE ENHANCEMENT
Words from the Wise:
Johanna Hedman, Board Certified Microblading Technician

Lip blushing is excellent from an anti-aging perspective. As we age, a lot of times we'll lose the definition around the contour of the lips, and we see a bit of wrinkles there. Lip blushing gives the illusion of full lips by going to the end of where you have lip tissue and extending the contours where you naturally have lifts. We do this very light where you can't really see it, so it helps a lot to make the lift look a little fuller. That way it brings a little more color to your face. Some clients want to go a little more intense and do a lipstick effect, though most clients want something natural where they wake up and it just looks like when they were eighteen or nineteen years old, when they had a naturally fresh glow and blush tone.

When you apply eye makeup, it's hard to get the liner close to the lashes and it's also hard to get in between them. But when you do it, it looks so nice, and gives an extra intensity to the eye and makes the eyes look more defined. The eye enhancement service allows us to do that for you in a more permanent way. We go in and get really close in between and above the eyelashes, and it will look like you have eyeliner on all the time. It will also give the appearance of fuller, darker eyelashes because of where the color sits at the base of the lashes. We can do this on the top and bottom lashes. It looks really polished and put together. You can also create a little wing for a bit of a cat eye look, though we don't do that a lot because it doesn't age very well over time (and because the skin by the eyes there often starts sagging over time and eventually it won't look good). All of this helps you feel very put together when you wake up. When I started in this business, I had two small kids and no time to do my eyebrows, eyes, and lips. Now, I just wake up, put on a little bit of foundation, a little blush, and I'm good to go, versus having to start from scratch. You save yourself time and you just feel better about yourself.

The use of micropigmentation can also go beyond makeup. We can use the tool to help camouflage scars as well, like scars people might have from surgeries. We find a color that matches the exact hue of the person's skin color and shade over the scar. It's very effective.

Permanent makeup is such a time-saver, and it looks freakin' gorgeous, so I definitely recommend it. Plus, you'll be glowing! (But, again, this doesn't mean you need to throw away your brow pencil, or lip color, or eyeliner though. I have my eyebrows and lips done, but I still take about three seconds every morning to put a little bit of extra makeup on. But it's so easy because I already have the shape. It's very simple to maintain.)

Wake Up Feeling Pretty

With permanent makeup, you can easily wake up every morning feeling like the prettiest version of yourself. And lashes can help bring it to the next level! Let's quickly start with strip lashes. Here is the process my close friend Monica Hart calls the "No-Fail Strip Lash Application."

What you'll need:
- Invisiband strip lashes
- Eyelash curler
- Clear eyeliner-style lash adhesive (Kiss is a good brand)
- Brush-on clear lash adhesive
- Spoolie
- Mascara

1. Curl lashes with an eyelash curler. This keeps straight lashes from sticking out and blends your natural lashes into the strip lashes.
2. Trim strip lashes with a small pair of eyebrow scissors. Only cut off lashes on the outer corners, never the inner. Trim off the little piece of extra band that sticks out on the inner corner,

avoiding cutting the short lashes. When trimming the outer lashes, only trim the excess. The lashes should cover your natural lash line and not extend past that.

3. Apply a generous coat of eyeliner-style eyelash glue to the upper lash rim, just above your natural lash line.

4. While that is drying a little bit, apply a generous (but not gloppy) amount of clear lash adhesive to the invisible band on the lashes. Only work with one strip at a time.

5. Using a pointed tweezer, gently grab a strip and apply the strip lashes to the appropriate eye. Apply them close to the base of the lashes, adjusting with the tweezer. The adhesive is still plenty wet, and the lashes can be moved to the correct position easily. Hold in place for a few seconds, making sure to hold corners down until less tacky.

6. Repeat for other eye.

7. Using the back end of a spoolie, tap across the entire rim of the lash band to ensure lashes are smooth and are lying flat. Repeat for other eye. Let dry for 30 seconds or so.

8. Lightly brush lashes with spoolie.

9. Finish by applying one light coat of mascara to the base of your natural lashes. This gives them lift and blends them into the strip lashes.

Once you're proficient, this process only takes 2-3 minutes or so per eye.

This is a good method for those who want to use strip lashes, but what about others who want long lashes but simply can't perfect that method? How do we achieve it? Well, there are, of course, various serums on the market that help eyelash growth, like Revitalash Advanced Eyelash Conditioner ($59) that you apply above the lash line once a day. I have friends who swear by this product!

But if strips and serums aren't right for you, another option (and one I personally use) is eyelash extensions. I go to Gisell Carrasco at Tres Chic Beauty Bar here in Miami (www.treschicbeautybar.com) to make my lashes look amazing, and she nails it every time. She's taught me a lot about this art. Like, do you ever look at someone with eyelash extensions and they look like they're weighing that person's eyelids down? Like Janice from The Muppets! Well, that happens when the technician doesn't use the right lashes for the person's eye shape (when they do them simply *way too* long and heavy). Like, with round eyes, it makes sense to use lashes that elongate and add volume to create a more almond-shaped appearance. But for hooded eyes, that volume might not be as necessary, since your main goal is to extend and lift to open the eyes. With almond-shaped eyes, the volume and length will usually be added to the outer corners, specifically, to emphasize the natural shape of the eyes. I find it all fascinating!

Here's more of what Gisell had to say about eyelash extensions.

EYELASHES

Words from the Wise:
Gisell Carrasco,
Eyelash Extension Technician

Eyelash extensions have become very popular in recent years. They're great for anyone who wants a daily low-maintenance beauty routine (including pregnant women.) All of my new client appointments start with a consultation. I'll talk to them about what they're looking for while also considering factors like their eye shape, size, any corrective measures needed, and so on. I then map out a customized approach for them so that they leave with something that enhances their natural features rather than overpowering them. We also take this time to talk about potential allergies and sensitivities.

Then we get going. The length of the sessions varies but the process for the initial full set can take from two- to three-and-a-half hours. The refill sessions take between two and two-and-a-half hours. During the session, the client lays down in a nice, comfortable bed while we do the lashes. Some of my clients even use that time to get in a nice little beauty nap. The entire process is completely painless (and often relaxing!).

I always send my clients off with an aftercare regimen that helps with longevity and health of their lashes. I recommend using specialized lash shampoos (it is so important to keep the lashes clean. We all naturally have teeny tiny mites in our eyelashes, but for the ladies who don't properly cleanse—especially those who leave a lot of makeup on their eyes, it can get out of control, not to mention the bacteria that can build up. I've seen it all and trust me, it can get bad). I also tell them to avoid sleeping on their face, and to steer clear of steam and saunas, as well as to avoid excessive makeup application. Coming back for refills is significant in maintaining the health and uniformity of the eyelashes. Lashes, much like the hair on your head, grow at different rates and cycles. Therefore, refills are important to ensure the extensions remain cohesive and aligned with the natural lash growth.

The cost of eyelash extensions varies widely, with a full set ranging from $125 to $600, depending on factors such as location and the artist's expertise. Refill sessions typically cost between $150 and $175.

Other popular eyelash services are the eyelash lift and the eyelash tint. An eyelash lift is like a perm for your eyelashes. I use a solution on the eyelashes to curl them into the client's desired shape. The result is a lifted and more open-eyed look. The eyelash tint involves coloring the eyelashes to make them darker and more defined. The darker lashes that result from this give an illusion that the person is wearing mascara. Eyelash lifts are usually between $50 and $150, and eyelash tints usually range between $20 and $75.

As I've now said on repeat (sorry to beat a dead horse!) but I find all of this to be worth it. Enhancing your teeth (if you have the funds) and having a permanent makeup look can both really play a part in changing your face for the better. And who doesn't want a better-looking face? You wouldn't have picked up this book if you didn't.

CHAPTER FOUR

DON'T FEAR
THE NEEDLE

Now that we've conquered skincare, and the face as a whole, it's time to take things a step further. Yes, it's time to discuss needles (and not just those teeny, tiny microneedles we talked about in Chapter 2, or the microblading needles for your eyebrows). I'm talking Botox, fillers, and other treatments you can get from the med spa. I'm talking *injectables!* Let's learn what every grown woman should be asking for when she goes in for treatments.

The Big B: Botox

Cosmetic Botox (which is our focus—there are other medical uses, but that's for a whole different book) is a treatment that involves injecting a substance derived from a toxin into specific muscles of the face to reduce the appearance of wrinkles and fine lines. Botox works by temporarily paralyzing or relaxing the muscles it's injected into. It makes your face look younger—the GOAL!

I didn't start using Botox until I was in my mid-thirties, for two reasons. First, it wasn't readily available at every med spa or corner salon like it is today. And second, because I didn't really need it. It wasn't until my mid-thirties that I started to notice some serious "resting angry bitch face" or, my "elevens," the two lines above the bridge of my nose creased in a permanent squint or scowl. It was time to try this new thing called Botox, but my friends were worried about it. "What if it makes my face lopsided?" they asked. "What if it makes my eyebrows rise so high that I look permanently freaked out?"

Fortunately, none of that happened.

I'm guessing that if you've made it all the way to Chapter 4 in a book on anti-aging, you're no stranger to Botox. But in case you're unfamiliar with it, rest assured: It's one of the treatments I get that barely hurts. (I like to say, ***"If it doesn't hurt, it doesn't work!"*** But with wrinkle relaxers like Botox, that's not the case.) There is a needle, but you can barely feel it. The only thing that might freak out newbies is that there might be a few tiny, raised bumps where the needle enters…and there might be a teeny bit of blood… and you may hear a wee bit of crunching from the needle going in. That is all perfectly normal! The bumps disappear in a few hours. If you're new to Botox, don't expect to look years younger right away. Wait a full week (some providers say up to ten days) for the true results. If after that time, you don't think it did much, you can usually go back to your provider for more. I've done that plenty of times.

There are conflicting views out there about Botox and other wrinkle relaxers (like Dysport) since some people consider these drugs to be poison for our bodies. There are lots of arguments on both sides, but I will say that these treatments are FDA approved, so you don't need to be scared to get it if you think it's right for you. For me, I've gotten wrinkle relaxers less and less over time. Instead, I mostly focus on the other treatments, procedures, supplements (ahem—peptides!) and more that I talk about in this book to keep me looking young. As of right now, I get Dysport and only do it about once a year.

In this chapter you're going to hear from one of my injectors, Julia Franklyn, PA-C, from Plump in Miami (@injectablesbyjulia on Instagram). She'll discuss how long Botox lasts, but it never lasts very long for me, *maybe* two months maximum, whereas for most people it lasts three months. Turns out, my body simply metabolizes Botox quicker than the average person. (I learned from Julia that this can happen when a person is very physically active; the only downside I've found to being insanely regimented. It can also happen when someone's body starts to become immune to injectables, which could be the case for me too.) I'm not sure exactly when I made the switch, but at some point, an injector had me try Dysport and it lasted a lot longer for me—usually up to six months. I recommend trial and error, as well as a consultation with your injector, as you're figuring out what to use to banish your own wrinkles. (I'm, for sure, not a doctor!)

It's very important to find a qualified professional who is board certified (MD, DONP, or PA—depending on the state). Back when injectables were first gaining traction, it was common to go to a dermatologist or a plastic surgeon's office. Today, med spas have popped up everywhere offering Botox and other injectables too. Some of these med spas are good and have certified professionals injecting, and some, well, *suck*! This is why doing your due diligence is so important. Always look for someone who is well-trained, with experience, who is well-reviewed, and comes from a reputable place.

The right injector will be able to set realistic expectations with you on what the treatment will do—what its capabilities are—and what its limitations are, which you'll hear from Julia. (I mean, Botox isn't going to change your entire face, and it's also not going to be solely responsible for turning back the clock 20 years either.) I also suggest examining the injector themselves to see if their look is something you want too. If your injector's look *isn't right* to you for any reason, it could be a sign that they're not the right one for you to use. Why risk you looking like that too?

Since Botox was the first big wrinkle relaxer on the market, let's start with a professional's take on that, shall we? Here is Julia to explain all there is to know about Botox as a wrinkle-relaxing option.

BOTOX
WORDS FROM THE WISE:
JULIA FRANKLYN, PA-C

With new clients, I first get their medical history. I ask about prior treatments they've had on the face beyond injectables, including any surgeries. I then ask if they've ever had undesirable results of something that didn't go as planned. It's critical to get that history and feedback. If they're nursing or pregnant, they can't inject anything.

Then I give them what I refer to as "Botox 101" because I want them to be well-informed and be able to decide what's right for them. I let them know about the different FDA-approved areas for Botox. We then talk about the areas of their face that bother them. Usually, they want my opinion on what they should get. I try to get them to focus on the areas of their face that bother them and work around that, versus any areas I'd suggest for them. There are certain aesthetic standards we do go by, and objective numbers and ratios, but of course not everyone fits into one mold.

Everyone has their own aesthetic goals for themselves, and you have to make sure you're aligned with your injector. From my perspective, I don't think injectables should change the way you look (unless you have asymmetry or a medical condition where there's an actual problem to treat or fix). The ideal injections will complement your natural features and simply enhance your look.

On a rare occasion I'll have a new client come to me in their fifties and show me a picture of themselves in their thirties to try to copy, and I'm honest with them—there is absolutely nothing you can do to get that exact look with that age difference. I try to educate them on graceful aging and knowing what looks appropriate for their age. Botox freezes the wrinkles, yes, but you're simply not going to look like you did five years ago or ten years ago, especially if you're an older patient.

The three most common areas that people get Botox are the frontalis (your forehead area), the glabella (the collection of muscles in between your eyebrows), and the crow's feet which are around the eyes. Botox cosmetic is FDA-approved for all three of those areas—though we do use Botox off-label all the time for the full face, as well as the neck and many other areas of the body. We can also treat the lower part of the face (like the corners of the mouth that can tend to pull the mouth down as you age) as well as the neck and the nose (to give the illusion of a slimmer nose). We also remind patients not to forget their hands either which can show signs of aging.

Sixty-four units is the FDA-approved dosing on Botox—20 units in the forehead, 20 units in between the eyebrows, and 12 and 12 around the eyes, though it's very common for people to get less. Of course, everyone has different muscle sizes, so it's always best to have a trusted injector help guide you in how much to get. Botox prices range quite a bit and can usually be somewhere between $10 and $18 per unit. I always tell people, if you don't have enough money to pay for the right number of units you need, save up until you do. It would be like needing a whole house painted and only having the funds to afford one can of paint. You wouldn't start painting until you could paint the whole thing, right?

For the first-time patient coming in though, I typically focus on the upper face with them, unless they have a specific concern in the lower face. That said, if someone older comes in for the first time, I might recommend beginning with everything because we're trying to play catch up.

There can be negative side effects of Botox, depending on the person, including things like swelling at the injection site and headaches. In regard to appearance, there is always a chance of an Artois of the brow or Artois of the eyelid where the eyelids can look almost like they're closed. If this happens, time is unfortunately the only cure, and the patient would have to wait until the Botox completely wears off.

Something people like about wrinkle relaxers is there's basically no downtime. The injector usually tells you to not exercise or lay flat for four hours, which is the amount of time it takes for the product to settle where it's supposed to go. They also say no facials or face massages for four hours too. It usually takes about two weeks for wrinkle relaxers to fully settle in, and then the four-to-six-week point will be the sweet spot, it's the tightest it will be, with the least amount of movement and wrinkles. Unless their body metabolizes it very fast like mine does, for most people Botox will last about three months, which is great for the cost when you think about it!

BOTOX
WORDS FROM THE WISE:
JULIA FRANKLYN, PA-C

So, when should you start getting Botox? I recommend patients start when they notice something that bothers them on their face. If one morning you wake up and start to see lines that are bothersome, start your research to find the right injector. Likewise, even if you're older, if certain lines on your face don't bother you, don't feel the pressure to do something about those.

I personally don't like to assess the start time by age. I recently had one client who was nineteen or twenty and she had a line in her glabella area when she frowned, so we took care of it. But I've had other women come in in their forties and there's not a single line on their face. Everyone ages differently due to things like genetics, sun exposure, lifestyle habits and so on. All these things play into what lines and wrinkles are on your face.

We always say in this world, it's easier to start with prevention than treatment. If you have a fine line that begins to form and you notice animation or motion you don't like, maybe the lines are there "at rest" but not fully or deeply ingrained—that's usually an appropriate time to start, as those lines are starting to set in and they're only going to get worse and harder to treat. I would say for the most part, most of my clients come in when the lines are starting to settle at rest and they want to prevent them from getting deeper, and that is truly different for everyone I have.

What I say is, if there is nothing at rest, my patients can wait. If there's no reason to treat, there's no reason to treat, right?

I love learning from Julia. When I hear certain rumors about Botox or Dysport—then she'll be right there to correct me. One common misconception is that Botox can fully lift your eyebrows. (The only thing that can *really* lift your eyebrows fully is surgery… I'm sorry to break it to you!) The truth as I've found from Julia is—the eyebrows sit where they sit. There's very little Botox can do to lift them, other than lifting the tail of the brow (meaning the outer most lateral portion). So, if you go to your injector, hold up the middle of your eyebrow to arch it, and tell them you want Botox to create that arch from an injection there in the forehead, it's not going to happen. Turns out, injecting actually *lowers* the brow there. Who would have thought? Thanks, Julia!

Dysport or Die

Another injector I frequently visit in Miami is Denise Santoli. She's another miracle worker, and always seems to know the right thing to recommend to keep my face looking taut and young. Since I've now switched from Botox to Dysport, I've learned a ton from Denise about the injectable.

Here are some quick facts about Dysport:

- **Injection areas:** Dysport is injected in the same areas as Botox, with the forehead, glabellar lines, and crow's feet as popular treatment spots.
- **Units needed:** It'll depend on the person, but usually people get between 20-80 units in their forehead, 40-80 in the eleven lines, and 15-30 units in the crow's feet.
- **Cost:** Units on average cost between $4 and $8 each.
- **How long it lasts:** Dysport usually lasts between three and six months, depending on the

person. The peak effect is usually within two weeks of treatment.

Here's Denise's take on Dysport for anyone considering going that route.

DYSPORT

Words from the Wise:
Denise Santoli, Injector

Dysport is a great alternative to Botox to relax wrinkles and help your face look younger. Dysport, like Botox, is a neurotoxin, but unlike Botox it's formulated differently. A lot of people who use it say they experience a faster onset of results and longer-lasting results. When it's injected, Dysport has a tendency to spread further, covering more area than a Botox injection would. For that reason, I recommend my clients go for Botox in cases when we're trying to treat a very specific purpose and area. Botox in those instances offers more control.

For new patients, particularly those in their thirties seeking to address forehead lines, I usually lean towards recommending Botox. After a while, our bodies start to metabolize Botox more quickly, and this is when I see patients often make the switch to Dysport. There are other alternatives to Dysport and Botox, like Daxxify, but I have reservations about how well they work and how long they last.

Lately, I've gotten a lot of requests for the "lip flip," and some of my patients have great results with it. The lip flip is done by putting wrinkle relaxer injections—either Botox or Dysport—directly above the line of the upper lip to give the lip a shape that appears fuller. It only takes a few units to do, and the results last the same amount of time as Botox or Dysport would elsewhere in the face.

Regardless of which wrinkle relaxer you go with, it's important to share your concerns with your injector, but also to listen to their recommendations. I always recommend a holistic approach to injections to make sure all of the problem areas are treated while preventing imbalances in facial movement. For example, there's a probability that if you neglect certain areas when getting injections then those untreated areas can start to show exaggerated movement that you otherwise wouldn't have noticed. To get the most natural and even look, you'll want your injector to help you address all problem areas.

Whether you land on Botox or Dysport, you're in good hands, as both are very effective. Just make sure you're following the sound advice myself and the experts have said endlessly throughout this book and be sure to go to someone who is an actual expert in this. Don't let yourself be tempted by that very cheap Groupon deal for Botox. We know better at this point.

A Little Plump Here, A Little Fill There…

Now, let's do a dive deep into fillers. I'm sure you already have some questions swirling for me (well, me *and* Julia). What is the best way to get rid of fine smoker lines? What about Kylie Jenner lips—should older women stay away from those? If so, why? What should you NOT do when it comes to lips? What is the best way to keep your lips looking natural?

Let's start with a definition. Fillers are substances injected into the skin to add volume and reduce the appearance of wrinkles or lines on the face and to create a smoother and more youthful appearance. They can also be used to plump up certain facial features, like the lips or cheeks.

Basically, when it comes to the face, while Botox and Dysport reduce wrinkles by relaxing the muscles, fillers reduce the appearance of wrinkles by plumping up the skin. The combination, when done correctly, can be a really flawless look. (It's very common for people to overdo the filler, though. That's why it's so important to go to a trained professional who has plenty of good reviews.)

Fillers are a go-to injectable for me, and honestly, I've gotten them almost everywhere at this point. Let's see: Lips, smile lines, chin, jaw, temples, nose, cheeks, knees, vagina, butt, hands, earlobes, corners of the mouth…I'm probably missing something, but that's a good summary. (You might be interested to know the nose fillers hurt *way more* than the ones in my vagina. The nose is *so sensitive!*)

I started with my lips many moons ago. The first time was a disaster, and my lips came out HORRIBLE! I looked like a duck. I swear this guy used two full syringes on my lips alone (if that means nothing to you, it will soon). I remember we were heading on vacation to Cabo

San Lucas, Mexico the next day. On the plane I kept wrapping a scarf around my face to hide. It was mortifying. Luckily, fillers can be dissolved, so that's what I did the second we got home. *"I'm never getting filler in my lips again!"* I declared to everyone who would listen.

Hah!

Once I eventually got them done the right way, it was a whole other world! I loved it so much that I couldn't even imagine my lips going back to the smaller shape they were before. I've personally only ever had one other bad side effect from filler after that initial duck lip scenario, and that was when I got a Y Lift (NEVER AGAIN) but more on that in the next chapter.

For me, filler usually lasts about four months though I've talked to some people who say theirs has lasted up to TWO YEARS! That's crazy! And no matter where I get the injections, it always looks great. Here's Julia's take on fillers, and more on current pricing.

FILLERS
Words from the Wise:
Julia Franklyn, PA-C

With filler, I follow a similar process with my new clients as I do with Botox. I start by going through their medical history and I find out what they've done in the past. Then, I hand them a mirror and ask what bothers them, then we get into the consult and communication and education. A lot of times clients explain what they want fixed with filler is not the actual thing they want fixed. We go through their concerns, and I explain what the appropriate fixes would be.

When it comes to filler, there has been a major shift toward full facial balancing. This means putting a little bit of filler everywhere as opposed to treating one thing. But a lot of times someone will come in and they just want to get their lips done, or their cheeks done, or a little filler here or there for certain lines. Sometimes that is appropriate, but sometimes I need to talk to them about the overall picture—the aesthetic standards and ratios and golden standards.

In Miami, I have a lot—and I mean a lot—of people who like to fill their lips, but you can imagine that eventually it's going to look disproportionate and abnormal compared to the rest of their face. Like I said, with Botox, the goal is not to make the person look like someone else completely new, but instead to make them feel refreshed and real while replacing lost volume.

As we age, we lose a lot of fat, but we also lose a lot of bone mass too. Because we don't have that mass to hold everything up, it all starts to drop. Usually for my older clients it's the lower part of their face that bothers them and they don't even see the mid-face, but I always recommend they treat top to bottom. I usually like to treat lateral to medial because that will end up using less product in the lower face when you replace the lost volume in the midface. This works excellent since everyone's goal is to always use as few syringes as possible for cost reasons.

One syringe of filler is equal to just one teaspoon, so it's a very small amount. When you're spreading that amount everywhere, it's not even noticeable. I usually start with anywhere from two to four syringes, and then I like to see my clients for a follow up usually every four weeks or so and we do a slow, gradual build until they get their desired results. From there, it can be maintenance, which is usually just one or two syringes per year. For lips, it's less, and I'll usually use one syringe maximum.

The biggest risk with filler is going to be vascular occlusion. It's rare, but it does happen. Vascular occlusion is when a vessel in the face is compromised—either by actual filler getting into the vessel or filler compressing it from pressure outside of the vessel. The blockage prevents blood from perfusing the area as it normally does. It can cause sudden pain, swelling, and changes to the skin color. And if you've heard of blindness with filler, it's the same idea as that—in that case you're blocking off the blood supply to the optic nerve and your eyesight can go black.

Some vascular occlusions are reversible, and some are not. I always educate my patients on the warning signs, which are those symptoms I just mentioned. I give my filler clients my contact information in the rare case it <u>did</u> happen so I could meet them in the clinic. I've never had to, but I would come into the clinic overnight if I needed to for an emergency. We don't tend to think about emergencies in esthetics, but they do happen on that very rare occasion. Other risks are far less serious, like bruising and swelling, especially with lip filler, and it often depends on how easily the person bruises.

The good thing about filler is that it's 100 percent reversible (when it's hyaluronic acid, dermal fillers). They're reversible with an enzyme called Hylenex. So, if for some reason you have any other complication or an undesirable result, it can be reversed.

Overfilling is another potential risk and can be a huge issue, cosmetically, for patients. All injectors should know better—just because a client wants more and more filler, does not mean they need it. We have a responsibility to make sure our clients don't go overboard. This is where it's important not to let the client sit in the driver's seat and get whatever they "think" they want. It's our job to help them keep things balanced and looking appropriate at the end of the day. I never fear telling a client "no."

We can do filler for clients in most places. One spot we often get requests for that can be touch and go, though, is the undereye. The undereye is a common complaint women have with their appearance and filler is effective in helping, but only for the right candidate. For the right candidate, it can be life changing, as it can alter the whole look of their mid-face and help them look more rested and refreshed. But again, not everyone is a good fit for this, so if you're considering undereye filler, definitely talk to your injector first. As with all areas of the body, it should be done on a case-by-case basis, and that area should always be under-corrected versus overfilled, because it is the most finicky area to fill.

As for filler for sagging jowls, that can certainly be helpful, again depending on the patient, and the degree of skin laxity. If the sag is significant, the filler can buy you maybe a couple of years, but in the end you're going to have to do something surgical.

One question my friends ask is: *"What do I do about my smile lines?"* Well, by the blessing of Julia and filler, I don't have them because we use a special technique. Julia uses a cannula on me; it's a tool that is longer than the usual injection tool, and it goes very deep into the tissues in my cheeks to deposit the filler. If we didn't go that deep, it wouldn't have the same positive effect on my smile lines. Trust me… ask your injector to use a cannula if they have it for smile lines! (And if your smile lines are noticeable, *and* you're a smoker, PLEASE STOP SMOKING!!)

So, what about the cost? Filler can usually range from about $500 to $1,500 for a syringe. Usually, the injectors will offer half syringe options as well, for people who don't need a whole lot. (I especially love Plump where Julia works because they'll even sell down to a ¼ syringe—really great for people who don't want to waste the filler and the money!) Keep in mind, if you think the deal you've found on filler is almost *too good,* chances are the injector offering the deal isn't the best. I'll leave it up to you whether you want to risk it, but just…*beware.*

As I've mentioned, I've gotten filler nearly everywhere. It's helped with wrinkles on my face, to plump my lips, to balance my face, to slim the shape of my nose and straighten it (Denise did this for me and it's one of the greatest things ever!), to enhance the appearance of my vagina, to fill in cellulite on my butt, to give my knees a more youthful look (who likes saggy knees?! *Definitely not me!)*, to help my hands look younger (hands are a HUGE sign of aging in women, as you likely know), and so much more. If you think a spot on your body could benefit from filler, just ask your trusted injector. They'll know what to do!

They'll also be able to guide you in what specific type of filler to use. Juvéderm, Restylane (great for hands in my experience), Radiesse (great for the butt in my experience), Renuva (it helps boost your body's own fat production in areas you've had age-related fat loss; in my opinion it's fine for small areas) and Sculptra are common ones you'll see. The only one I've highly regretted getting was Sculptra which stimulates collagen production. That seems like a good thing, right? Well, sometimes this stimulation of collagen can leave behind granulomas, which are little unsightly nodules on the skin near the injection site. Aftercare for Sculptra involves regularly massaging the treatment area (this is unique to Sculptra, so please consult with your injector before massaging filler injection sites), but even though I did this as directed, and despite these nodules being a fairly rare side effect, it still happened to me. Now I have to use CO2 laser treatments to remove the scarring left behind from this experience.

Again, finding the right injector for fillers is the best path to ensure you won't look overdone or puffed up (like some of those women you might *eeeekkk!* at who've taken it too far). If it's not done right, it can totally change the shape of your face—in a terrible way. If the goal is to look natural, find an injector who looks natural too. Look at the before-and-afters of her patients to see if they look natural. Start with less and then build up to more, as needed. Ask your partner how you look…they'll be honest (mine always is)! The goal here is to have a fresh, youthful looking face, not to look like you just got stung by a thousand angry bees. Put it this way: If you think you've gone too far, chances are, you probably have.

Lifting It All Up with Threads

While they're not injections as this chapter aims to focus on, I want to spend a few minutes talking about threads, which are an alternative to filler and a non-surgical alternative to a facelift. So, what are threads? They're basically exactly what they sound like. If there's an area of your face or body that needs lifting, threads are a minimally invasive way to do it. Dissolvable threads are inserted under the skin and then used to lift and tighten the sagging areas. The results are usually kind of subtle (compared to something like a facelift, for example, where the results are *spectacular*—I'm obsessed with my facelift, which we'll get to) but there isn't any downtime (huge bonus!) and they can last up to three years when done properly. The results are immediate (huge bonus #2!), and another great thing is that the threads themselves stimulate collagen production.

I've had varied experiences with threads when it comes to my face (more on this in the next chapter). Since I never consistently loved my results, I made a firm and bold declaration: *I, San-*

dy Silverman, HATE threads for the face! But then during a recent visit with Denise, my mindset was changed completely. She did a couple of threads for me to tighten and lift parts of my face and neck that seemed a little too droopy for my liking, and now I've retracted my ban! Denise is now the only one I'll trust to do threads in my face.

Denise also does threads for me in other areas of my body, too, like my neck (the results are amazing!) and my knees. I did the threads in my knees a few years ago and I was blown away by how much younger my knees looked (knees are an area of the body that can really speak to a person's age, so having non-wrinkly knees made me very happy!). Knee threads, and threads in the neck, stomach, and elsewhere in the body, can be incredibly painful, I won't lie to you, but the results can be great when done by the right professional.

Since Denise is the one with all the knowledge on this topic, here is her take on threads, how they are used, and why they're worth it.

THREADS

Words from the Wise:
Denise Santoli, Injector

Threads are dissolvable sutures used to lift and reposition the skin, helping people look younger. This procedure is particularly popular for people who want a subtle facial rejuvenation without the downtime and risks associated with a facelift. Threads can be very helpful in addressing concerns on the face. They can be used to outline the mouth for more defined borders and to help with accordion lines. They can be used on other places on the body too to help with body contouring. Think of the places we tend to see loose skin as we age, like arms, elbows, stomach, and knees. I love using threads for clients with sagging skin on their necks too. Instead of using Botox there, which can be costly (usually more than sixty units are needed for the neck) and has results that fade within a couple of months, the threads give a tighter look that lasts longer. Threads in the neck will also leave a smoother, firmer appearance than you would get with Botox.

I start with my clients with a consultation where we talk about their aesthetic goals. During the actual thread lift procedure, the patient is awake and under local anesthesia. I'll strategically insert thin threads made of absorbable materials, such as polydioxanone (PDO), into the skin through small incisions. These threads have tiny cones or barbs that grip the underlying tissues and lift them upward when tension is applied.

Once the threads are inserted, I'll gently pull the threads to lift and reposition the skin as needed. The number of threads I'll use on the client and the placement of the threads depends on the patient's unique anatomy and the results they're looking for. The entire procedure usually takes about thirty to sixty minutes to complete, making it a convenient option for individuals with busy lifestyles too. In and out!

Pain should be minimal for the patient if the threads are done correctly. Every patient is different, and so will tolerate the pain differently, but for the most part, there usually isn't much discomfort for facial threads. After the thread lift procedure, patients might have some swelling, bruising, and mild discomfort, but these symptoms will typically subside within a few days. I tell my clients to avoid strenuous activities, refrain from excessive facial movements, sleep with their head elevated to minimize swelling, apply ice as needed, and take Arnica (an over-the-counter remedy) as needed to prevent and help with bruising. I also tell them to avoid touching or rubbing the treated area and to use gentle skincare products (which should also be applied gently).

Results from threads are noticeable right away after the procedure, but the full effects become more obvious when the swelling subsides, and the threads settle into place. The results are temporary, but can last up to three years, which is an impressive amount of time considering how minimally invasive they are, and how simple the procedure is. Plus, over time, although the threads begin to dissolve, the extra collagen they promote remains. Another big benefit with threads is that there is no scarring at all, like you'd experience with surgical options for tightening skin.

The cost can vary a lot depending on the experience of the person doing the procedure and how many threads are needed. On average, for threads in the face, on the low end I would say to expect to pay about $1,500, and on the high end it can be about $4,500. Threads can be complicated to do, much more so than the injectables, so you really need to make sure you're going to someone who knows how to do them properly. This is where you'd definitely want to prioritize expertise over cost. If you see threads offered for a very low price—let's say something like $200—steer clear. Don't compromise quality on something like this, because there are risks, and your results can be terrible if you go to the wrong person. (Just ask Sandy!) Don't rely on discounts, and instead focus on finding a reputable practitioner who can deliver consistent and safe results—results you're actually very happy with.

Let's Look on the Brightside: SKINVIVE

Professional brightening treatments for your face can make a real difference in getting super glowy, *"Look at her!"* type skin. SKINVIVE is a popular treatment and was created by the same company known for its fillers: Juvéderm. It's injected into the skin to give long-term hydration and radiance.

It also promotes firmness. With regular use, it can improve skin texture, reduce the appearance of fine lines and wrinkles, and enhance overall skin health. It's usually done through two injections of microdroplets directly into the face, and the injector will numb the injection spots ahead of time to help with any potential discomfort.

I tried SKINVIVE for the first time while writing this book, and let me tell you, my face was freaking *glowing.* I almost couldn't believe the results I got from it. I had people coming up to me for days after I got it asking what I'd done to get my skin to look so radiant and I was excited to tell them all about this new product. It's supposed to last up to six months, and for me, it's definitely met that expectation.

For the two injections, SKINVIVE usually costs between $650 and $750. I'd recommend having a conversation with your injector to see if it's a fit for you before you try it. (Like, my injector, Denise, told me, it's good for brightening and smoothing out little, fine lines, but won't have the same positive effect on someone with deeper lines.)

All of these are worth considering if you're ready for some pokes and injections but aren't ready for surgery just yet. Whether it's Botox, filler, threads, a skin brightening treatment, or any injectable, you have to find a trusted professional and together figure out what's right for you and your specific needs…and your wallet, too! I get that all of this can get expensive, so if you can't afford everything you want, you just have to prioritize. And if you're never ready for the surgical route, that's more than okay! Everyone is different.

I'll discuss this more in the next chapter, but one thing I do recommend if you're on the fence about surgery is this: If you're contemplating a facelift, do it sooner rather than later, like in your early forties. Experts agree on this for reasons we'll soon get into, and my *only regret* about having my face lift in my late forties is that I didn't get it sooner. But if there is no way surgery is for you, read along for the next few chapters anyway—I have some entertaining stories to share!

CHAPTER FIVE

CHANGING FACES

In a shocking revelation to no one…I've never shied away from plastic surgeries. I'd like to tell you I was scared to take the leap into surgery, to help ease any of your own fears. To make you feel like, *"Oh, well Sandy's been there, and she got through the nerves!"* But I'd be lying.

I'm sorry.

Looking my best has forever been the goal, and as long as I wasn't totally breaking the bank, I knew I'd be game to try anything. I honestly can't remember a time I felt intimidated to go under, even back in my twenties. That's when I felt that first itch, and I *needed* to scratch it. One day I looked in my mirror and thought, "Sandy, you need bigger boobs!" (We'll talk more about *the ladies* in the next chapter.) Around the same time, I also got my first nose job (yes, there have been multiple nose jobs). Again, I went in fearless, and even though it was a *bit* of a disaster (pun intended, as that plastic surgeon's signature style was *ittty bitty* noses), I didn't give up hope. I knew that, through the right surgeries, I could obtain—and sustain—the hottest version of myself humanly possible.

I've had *so many* surgeries since my twenties and I've been very happy with (nearly) all of them—most of all, my facelift! My facelift is, hands down, the best thing I've ever done. If you're like me, and most women over forty, you've probably looked in the mirror and envisioned how your face might look if the skin was a little tauter, or if your chin was tucked up just a tad. And I mean not just softer or smoother a la creams and lotions, but well beyond what products, injectables, and threads can do. Maybe after this self-examination in the mirror, you then immediately Google for this "miracle" serum or that "tighten it all!" tool.

But as Mindy Kim told us all the way back in Chapter 1, no products are truly miracles—though they may help, of course. I spent four chapters brain-dumping about the many things you can do to improve your face and skin before surgery, and I fully stand by everything I wrote. But as our bodies age and our skin starts to take the downward plunge, it's very hard to fix the sag without surgery.

And that, my friends, is the cold hard truth: Our skin will sag as we age—even if we've done everything else right.

Now, I realize not *everyone* will want or need a facelift. I fully support whatever decision you make! If you prefer to embrace the natural aging process, then let nothing stand in your way. But if that sag is getting you down, then please…allow me.

There's only one way to turn that frown literally upside-down and achieve a sag-free face—and that's by a facelift. For anyone unfamiliar with what that entails, a facelift is a surgical cosmetic procedure that lifts and pulls the facial skin so that it is taut. It tightens the skin on the face and neck to reduce wrinkles, sagging, and other signs of aging. By removing any excess skin and repositioning the tissues, a facelift helps achieve a smoother, more youthful appearance. Sag, be gone!

But you may be thinking, "Sandy, what about the pain? How do I even start to sift through the many options? And what about the freakin' *cost?!*"

Yes, there's plenty to consider, but first let's calm that anxiety. If you want a facelift, then don't let nerves about the surgery intimidate you. The biggest way to squash this fear—no matter what plastic surgery you're considering—is to: Do. Your. Research! And I'm not talking about a quick Google search, either. Take the time to read through plastic surgeon websites, and make sure you focus on plastic surgeons who *specialize* in facelifts. That part is so important. There are endless plastic surgeons out there who seem to do it all, but I highly recommend making sure you go to someone who is known for their facelifts. Then spend even more time reading through reviews from their patients. If reviews mattered for other treatments and procedures we talked about earlier in the book, they matter even more with surgery!

Check if the plastic surgeon has a social media presence and then scroll through it to preview their work. The more research you do, the more likely you are to find the right surgeon—and the more comfortable you'll feel heading into the process.

A lot of what holds people back from surgery is, well, it's *surgery.* You might be thinking, "Why would I *choose* to get surgery? Why would I put myself in this position?" Well, if it's something you really want, then it's worth it. And if you've done the deep research to find the right surgeon, fear not.

But I get it; many people get a pit in the bottom of their stomach even *thinking* about anesthesia, or potential surgical complications, or the recovery process. But finding a great surgeon means you're in great hands all around. When you pick the right one, be honest with them about your fears. Remember: They've performed this surgery hundreds of times, if not more. The right surgeon will have the answers to all your questions and will know exactly what to say to assuage your fears and calm you the heck down. Then, all you'll have to focus on is how absolutely stunning and youthful you'll look once you've healed.

Is there a stigma associated with plastic surgery? Yeah, there is and sometimes this is where the nerves associated with plastic surgery come from. People worry what their friends, family, coworkers—and anyone else—will say once they discover they've gotten a facelift (or any other cosmetic surgery). Well, you know what…f*ck them!

Listen: Everyone is unique. It's perfectly fine to want to look the way you want, whether that's aging naturally or exploring options that help you feel—and look—younger. And really, *WHO CARES?* Why should anyone care what you or anyone else is doing with their own body? Many, many people opt for cosmetic surgery procedures and the best plastic surgeons enjoy a thriving business with happy repeat customers. You're in plenty of good company, so kick your fear to the curb!

I've never kept secrets about the plastic surgery I've had done because…why add to that unnecessary stigma? Every day, I see women (and men) walking the streets of Miami with *perfect* faces and *perfect* bodies. I know there's more to their story.

But let's address the elephant in the room about why some women still tend to be so secretive about their choice: Because sometimes their significant other makes them feel judged for wanting to feel and look better by going under the knife. And this keeps women from getting the surgery they want.

WHY???!!!

Here's my take: If there is something—any-thing—*you* want to do to improve yourself, your partner shouldn't stop you. If you have the means to do it, then go for it. Making changes to your appearance, whether it's as simple as a new haircut, or as big as an elective surgery like a facelift, the decision should be up to you, and only you. We, as women, have a right to choose what is best for our own bodies! Personally, I want to be happy with all aspects of myself. And how can anyone be happy when they don't have the freedom they want?

That's why I will die on this hill—my facelift was the best thing I have *ever* done. It set me back decades. It was *life changing*. The only regret I have about my facelift is that I didn't do it sooner! The results are never going to be as good as they will be when you're younger, and experts agree, and I wish I did mine when I first wanted it in my early forties. So, if you're in your forties and considering it, I encourage you to go right away. Here's how my experience played out.

Me & My Facelift

I'll say it again, and even louder this time: I'VE NEVER LOVED A PROCEDURE AS MUCH AS I'VE LOVED MY FACELIFT. My journey to facelift bliss didn't start out that way, though.

One morning, at the ripe old age of forty-two, I woke up, looked in the mirror, and realized my face was literally sagging. Specifically, the skin around my lips seemed to change overnight. I stood there, lifting the skin with my index finger and letting go, over and over. I kept thinking, *What the Hell happened to my face?*

I decided right then that I wanted my skin to look tighter—and quickly (and permanently!). I wanted to look freakin' taut y'all, and I wanted those jowls and that double chin pulled way back. It was time to say, "See ya!" to all that droop and "Hello!" to the face of my youth. The answer: a facelift.

Of course, first I needed to find a doctor I could fully trust. But before I got very far in my research, my mom intervened, coming in 100 percent against the facelift idea. She practically begged me not to do it. I eventually gave in and agreed to pump the brakes on surgery and opted for a non-surgical option instead called the Y Lift.

I had heard about the Y Lift while watching *Good Morning America* on TV one morning. A doctor named Yan Trokel in New York City was talking about this new method he'd started practicing called the Y Lift. It was a minimally invasive procedure that used filler to lift and contour the face. I was glued to my chair listening to this guy talk.

According to Dr. Trokel, the Y Lift usually targets the cheekbones, the skin under the eyes, the jawline, and those marionette lines around the mouth for that lifted effect. It sounded like people who weren't quite ready for surgery loved it because there were no incisions and no downtime for recovery, just strategically placed fillers. The process was also super quick—it could be completed in about thirty minutes and the effects were immediate, whereas facelifts can take a few weeks to see any results. Plus, the effects were long-lasting, depending on how quickly your body metabolizes filler (discussed in Chapter 4). All in all, this sounded major! This was my chance to get the kind of tightening I was looking for while still listening to what my mama told me! I was ready for more volume and less sagging skin.

I made an appointment with Dr. Trokel quicker than you can say "tightening!" On the day of my appointment, I arrived, he injected me with filler for the Y Life, and I was out the same day with no downtime. And the results looked good…at least the first time around. My face definitely looked lifted, for a while, and I really liked the sculpted look.

But the next time I went back a few months later, the results were…awful. Dr. Trokel had used the cannula to go deep into the muscle in my face, particularly around my jawline. He plumped my face so badly that it looked like a *pie!* It was round and just awkward looking! In his defense, it was 2015, and that pie-faced look was sort of *in*—just not for me! So, by trying to keep up with whatever that trend was my face now looked horrible! It was a disaster.

At the time I'd gotten that second Y Lift, I was living in Miami. So, I tracked down a new plastic surgeon there to start the filler removal process. It took us forever to get all that filler out of my face. When we finally did, the plastic surgeon suggested threads to lift things. But she totally botched it! Whatever she did with the threads was nothing like how Denise Santoli does mine now. My face looked totally uneven, like someone had done a botched sewing job—which is *exactly* what had happened. Looking in the mirror made me cringe far more than it had before all of this began. (This is when I swore off face threads, before finally finding success with them through Denise.) I was frustrated, to say the least.

That's when I struck gold and found Dr. Leslie Baumann's office in Miami (www.derm.net; where Amy Koberling works). The threads started to slowly dissolve (all threads dissolve on their own over time) and the ladies at Dr. Baumann's office were able to get my face looking even again. But now I suddenly had *so much* sagging—much more than I'd ever had!

By now, it was 2018. I was forty-seven years old, and I seriously regretted not getting that facelift years earlier. I couldn't stop thinking about it. Finally, I made the decision to go down a rabbit hole of research on facelifts until I found the right doctor. It was time to take the leap to fight gravity once and for all!

But I knew if I was going to act on it, I needed to research, and research well. I started within my own social network, asking around to see what I could expect in terms of cost, but also… *Who was the best?*

In a traditional facelift, the surgery addresses the sagging areas on the face and neck. Once the patient is under anesthesia, the doctor will make incisions around the hairline to the ear (and possibly behind it and beneath it). The excess skin is then lifted, which in turn lifts the entire lower portion of the face with it. And the tissue beneath is tightened by cutting and removing the excess. This leaves the skin with a smooth and youthful appearance, which is a *dream come true* for those with advanced signs of aging.

All my research led me to Dr. Andrew Jacono in New York City (www.newyorkfacialplasticsurgery.com). If his name sounds familiar, that is because he is one of the best plastic surgeons in the country. I was beyond impressed with the before-and-afters on Dr. Jacono's website, so I scheduled a consultation, packed my bags, and flew to New York.

As soon as I started talking to Dr. Jacono during our consultation, I knew he was the doctor to perform my surgery. We talked through my many different options (who knew there were *so many* facelift options?!) and scheduled the procedure on the spot.

Despite getting knocked out (of course) for the procedure, the whole process seemed like no big deal. I was in and out in about three hours. After I left, my husband and I went straight to lunch at Freds at Barneys. (Granted, I was still drugged up, dopey, talking nonsense, and SO swollen…but we ate!) My recovery took a few weeks, exactly what I was told to expect, and while I was very swollen during that time, the recovery was easy otherwise. (Even after I fully healed, the puffiness remained which is why I eventually incorporated lymphatic work into my daily routine.) Personally, I found it easy to keep the swelling and bruising at bay by icing as much as possible and taking Arnica daily.

Dr. Jacono had knocked it out of the park. I looked a decade younger, if not more. Sometimes I look back on my own before-and-after images from that surgery and I still can't wrap my head around how good a job he did. If I hadn't gotten my facelift when I did, I would look soooo much older now. I wouldn't even want to walk out of my house looking like that—I'd be too miserable.

After my facelift, it's been no more nonsense for me. I stay on top of everything I do for my skin (as you now know from earlier chapters!) and treat it well. I remain totally cautious about who I go to for treatments and commit to only the best of the best people.

Facelifts usually need to be repeated every ten to fifteen years. I'm at the five-year mark as I'm writing this and I'm not sagging at all, which makes me really happy. But I'll definitely do it again when the time comes, and I won't go to anyone else but Dr. Jacono. He is on the more expensive side for sure (I believe his facelifts now cost upward of $250,000—yes, the same amount that, in some places in the country, would buy an entire home!), but he's worth every penny. Plus, he already knows my face, and what's best for it. Why go to anyone else?

On the topic of cost: Facelifts can run a huge range depending on the location and the doctor. I will say that if you find someone willing to do a facelift for less than $10,000, then it's probably a risk (please see my Y Lift story). One good thing is that many doctors allow payment in installments, which is a worthwhile option for those who might not have all of the money up front.

Yes, facelifts are expensive. For that reason alone, they may not be for everyone. But, as with anything else of value, if it's something you really want, consider setting aside a separate savings account and stashing away a few dollars here and there to save up for it.

Faces Age, That's Just a Fact!

One day I was in Amy Koberling's office for a CO2 laser appointment when I couldn't help but notice a flip book she had on the counter. The book showed images of the natural progression of how a woman's face ages and it was…CRAZY! As I flipped through, I cringed thinking of how my face might look if I hadn't been doing everything in my power to keep looking young—and especially if I hadn't gotten my facelift. But it's not just our skin that ages, it's the muscle *and* the bones beneath it!

The reality is, we can hope and pray, we can ask a genie to grant our wish not to age, but *we are going to age* anyway. There's no way around it. As we approach our forties, our body's natural production of collagen and elastin (the pro-

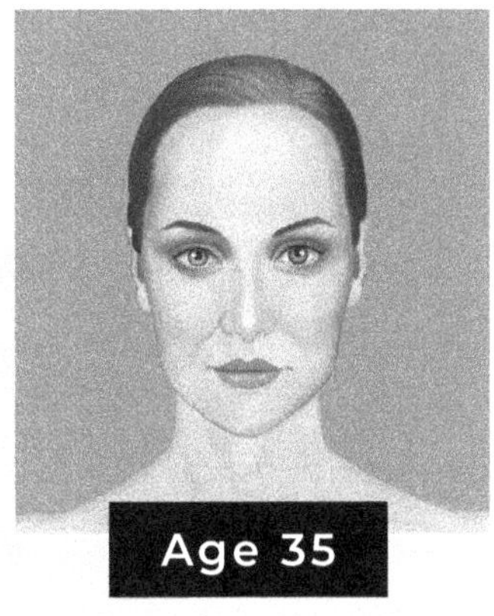

Facial aging is due to changes in several types of tissue including skin, fat, muscle, and bone. Changes in one tissue layer have an effect on the other layers.

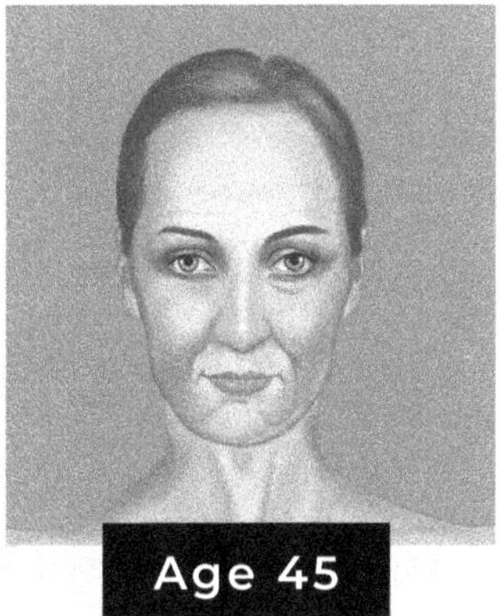

Skin

With age, skin undergoes several changes. Changes include:

- Thinner skin
- Skin more likely to wrinkle of sag
- Drier skin

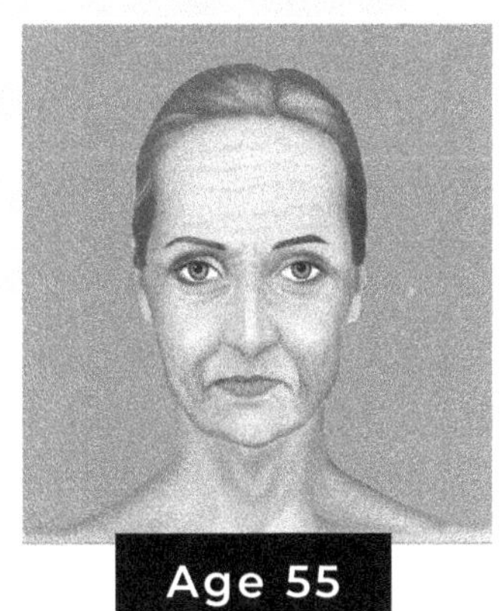

teins responsible for maintaining skin elasticity) decreases. Because of that, we will start to lose firmness and resilience in the skin, which results in sagging and drooping, particularly around the cheeks, jawline, and neck. The loss of collagen and elastin, combined with our old friend gravity, can lead to less definition along the jawline and the formation of the dreaded *jowls*. The skin and underlying tissues may sag, resulting in a less defined and youthful contour. (If you're unfamiliar with what jowls are, think of an older person whose skin around their jaw seems to sag lower than the jawbone. Those are jowls.)

Then, of course, there are the wrinkles and fine lines, which only seem to deepen by the day. By our forties and fifties, those wrinkles and lines become more pronounced than ever (UGH!). This is the age when we also start to lose volume in our faces as fat and muscles decline and this can result in a somewhat sunken look. We end up looking kind of sickly and exhausted.

Added to this is a decrease in cell turnover, which can change our skin texture and tone to become rougher and more uneven in appearance. And—gah!—then there's the age spots, the duller appearance of the skin as our natural exfoliation process slows. And our poor eyes—the delicate skin beneath the eyes is especially prone to aging, leaving us with puffy bags, dark circles, and hooded eyelids.

It's like *everything* is working against us! But then there's…

FACELIFT TO THE RESCUE! I realize this might sound like an advertisement for facelifts at this point, but in my opinion, it is the best way to turn back the clock on alllllllll of that aging nonsense. It helps tighten loose skin sagging everywhere, it reinstates those beautiful, youthful facial contours you used to have and love (talk about sculpting!), and it smooths out any pronounced wrinkles around the mouth, nose, and eyes--anywhere you're not already using wrinkle relaxers.

And, honestly, the confidence I felt after my facelift was unlike anything else. I may not have fully realized it before, but the way my face sagged was taking a toll on my emotional well-being! I didn't like the way I looked and that affected so many other parts of me. After the facelift, I felt like a completely different person.

Beyond the Norm: Other Types of Facelifts

I had always figured there was only one type of facelift—the traditional full surgical facelift that was tailored to an individual's specific face needs and concerns. And that was it. But during my own facelift journey, I learned there were many different types of facelifts beyond the traditional. Here are a few popular ones.

Mini Facelift:

A mini facelift offers a subtler change to the face, with more of a focus on the lower face and neck areas. It's performed similar to the traditional facelift, but with smaller incisions made only around the targeted areas of concern. It's super effective in smoothing out fine lines—think of it more as a "touch up." The mini facelift is also less expensive (prices usually are between $7,000 and $9,000) and, due to fewer incision sites, the overall recovery time is reduced, usually only about one to two weeks. This is often an ideal option for people with milder aging.

(It's great for ladies in their early forties!) Bonus: This procedure is often done with a local anesthesia (or twilight sedation) as opposed to general anesthesia.

Deep Plane:

A deep plane facelift targets the *deep plane* layer beneath the surface of the skin. As with a traditional facelift, the areas under the skin are treated; but the difference in a deep plane facelift is that the focus is on repositioning and lifting the muscles and fat pads underneath the skin. The procedure can target anywhere on the face or neck and is said to have a longer lasting effect than a traditional facelift. That said, it can also come with a bigger price tag (usually between $15,000 to $30,000) and a slightly longer recovery time, with bruising and swelling usually lasting three or more weeks.

Mid-Facelift:

A mid-facelift is for improvements on the middle region of the face, addressing sagging cheeks and nasolabial folds—making those cheekbones *pop* again like they did years ago. The process involves incisions typically made around the hairline and ears; this allows the surgeon to lift and reposition the underlying tissues. The recovery time is shorter than a traditional facelift and tends to be about a week or two. And the cost is less, too, and commonly goes for around $6,000 to $8,000.

SMAS Facelift:

The Superficial Musculoaponeurotic System (SMAS) facelift is a surgical technique that focuses on lifting and tightening the deeper layers of facial tissues. By addressing the SMAS layer—the layer that connects the skin and the deep tissue of the face—surgeons can achieve more significant, and longer-lasting results compared to traditional facelifts. This approach is often preferred for individuals with advanced aging concerns. Swelling and bruising usually lasts about a week. Costs for this can range pretty greatly—usually $8,000 and up.

Incision-less Facelifts:

For those looking for a non-surgical approach, liquid facelifts have emerged as an okay option. This technique uses injectables, such as dermal fillers and neurotoxins, to restore volume, reduce fine lines, and lift specific facial areas. The advantage lies in minimal downtime (usually only a couple of days) and the ability to achieve a more youthful appearance without the need for surgery. This option is also cheaper—it usually ranges from about $2,000 to $3,000.

And the future is upon us. As I'm writing this chapter, I just found out about another advancement in facelifts. And this one also involves exactly zero incisions. A stem cell facelift is done by first drawing your own blood and extracting stem cells, which are known for their regenerative properties. Then, your stem cells are injected in targeted areas of your face to stimulate collagen production, promote tissue regeneration, and improve skin texture. No scars! Virtually painless! But is it worth it? I guess as more patients try it, time will tell…Though for the $20,000+ price tag, I'm a bit skeptical.

The Risk of it All

Because we're talking about surgery here, I want to make sure you have a full picture of the procedure. This includes some of the following risks associated with getting any type of facelift (these apply to other plastic surgeries, so just take a mental note now):

- **Anesthesia:** There is always a risk going under, particularly with general anesthesia, such as allergic reactions and respiratory complications. Your surgeon will evaluate your medical history and overall health beforehand to determine the safest anesthesia approach.

- **Bleeding:** Bleeding during or after surgery is a potential risk of any facelift procedure—but it's rare. To minimize the risk of bleeding, it's important to follow your surgeon's pre-operative instructions and to avoid certain medications and supplements that can increase the risk of bleeding.

- **Infection:** As with any surgery, there is a risk of infection after a facelift. Your surgeon will take precautions to minimize this risk, such as administering antibiotics before-and-after surgery and maintaining strict sterile techniques during the procedure. However, if an infection does occur, it may require treatment with antibiotics or, in severe cases, surgical drainage.

- **Poor wound healing:** Some individuals may experience delayed wound healing or wound separation following a facelift, particularly if they have underlying medical conditions. Lifestyle factors such as smoking can also impair the body's ability to heal. Follow your surgeon's post-operative care instructions, including proper wound care, and avoid activities that strain the incision sites to help reduce the risk of wound healing complications.

- **Scarring:** All surgical procedures result in some degree of scarring, and facelift surgery is no exception. Your surgeon will make incisions in inconspicuous locations, such as along the hairline and behind the ears, to minimize visible scarring. However, individual scarring patterns can vary, and some individuals may experience more prominent or more visible scars than others.

- **Bad results:** Listen, it is possible—though unlikely—that you won't like your results. I can't stress this enough: Be crystal clear with your surgeon ahead of time about your goals and understand their take on realistic expectations. This can really make a huge difference in ensuring you're happy with your post-surgery look.

Always discuss any risks and concerns with your surgeon before making the decision to get any facelift. By carefully following their pre- and post-operative instructions, any risks will be minimized, leaving you with a safe experience—and *amazing* results.

A Quick Tip About Lip Lifts

Let's pause here for a quick, honorable mention in the overall category of *lifts*. When I started writing this book, I was just about to get a lip lift. I had a consultation with an excellent doctor in Miami that went well, and I was excited. Before I went in for the procedure, I had a regular visit with my injector, Denise Santoli. When I told her about my upcoming lip lift, she stopped me in my tracks.

A lip lift is done to enhance the upper lip—making it appear fuller and more youthful—by removing any excess skin between the lip and the nose, which shortens that distance. As we get older, the area between the nose and the upper lip naturally increases, so it's an obvious sign of aging. That said, the procedure leaves behind a younger appearance. It's also known to improve overall facial harmony. But, again, Denise tells me it's not for everyone. Here is Denise's take on why a lip lift might not be the answer.

LIP LIFTS
Words from the Wise:
Denise Santoli, Injector

I've had lots of clients come into my office to treat scars, so I know how long it can take to reduce them (often multiple laser treatments). That's why I'm always very honest with my clients if I think the scarring that will result from certain surgeries or procedures will be worth it. With lip lifts I'm very cautious. For someone with Sandy's lip shape—a full upper lip—and not too much distance between her nose and lip, the scar that would be left from a lip lift would not be worth it. Now, years down the road, when that distance between her nose and upper lip starts to increase more due to aging, this may be a different story, but for now I recommend against it. This is especially true when you consider the cost of a lip lift procedure, which can be around $10,000.

If you're someone who doesn't have a full upper lip and is interested in a lip lift, be sure to talk to a surgeon first and make sure it's right for you. And shop around. I was quoted $10,000, but you can definitely find this procedure in other parts of the country for less and with equally qualified surgeons.

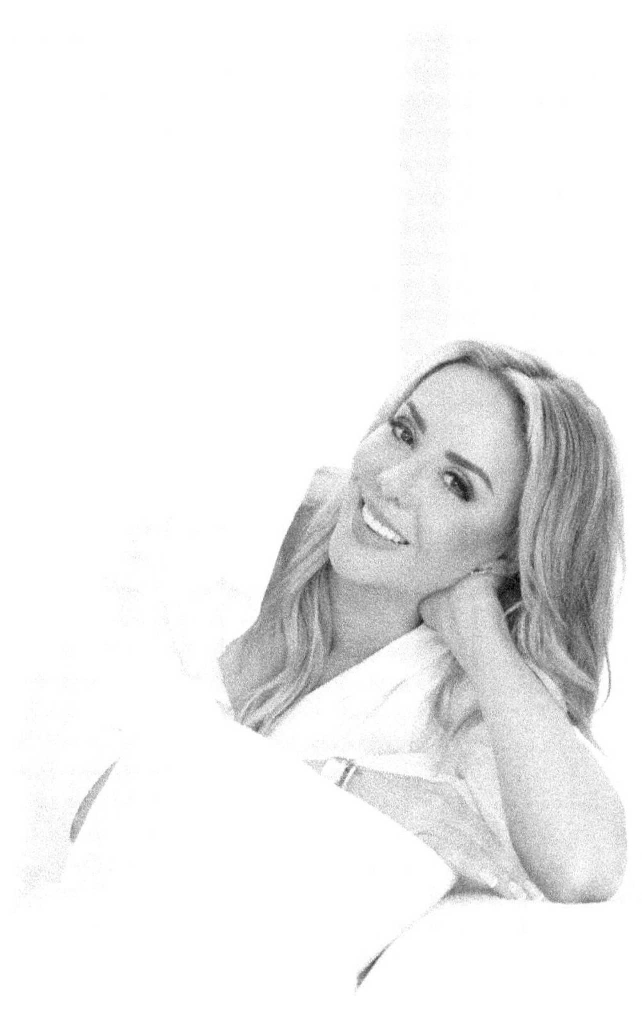

CHILDHOOD

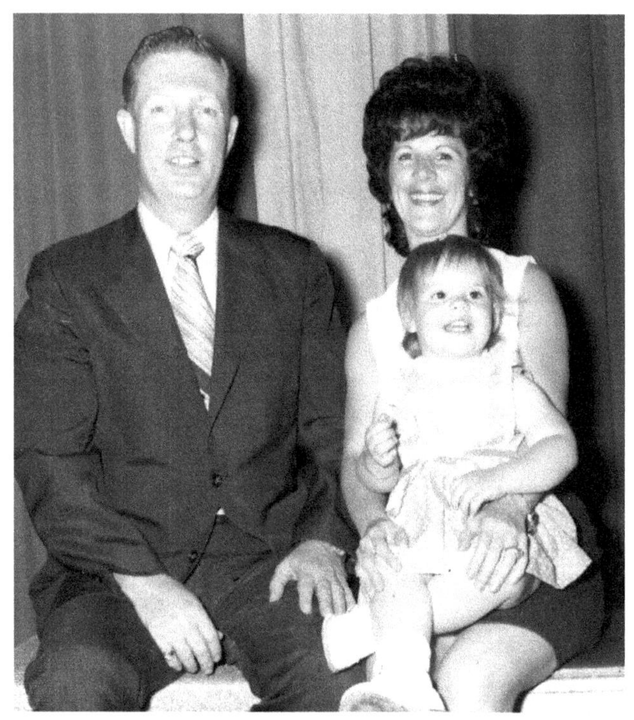

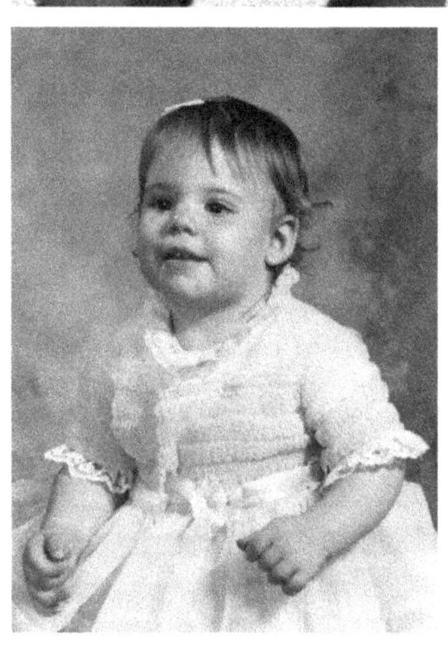

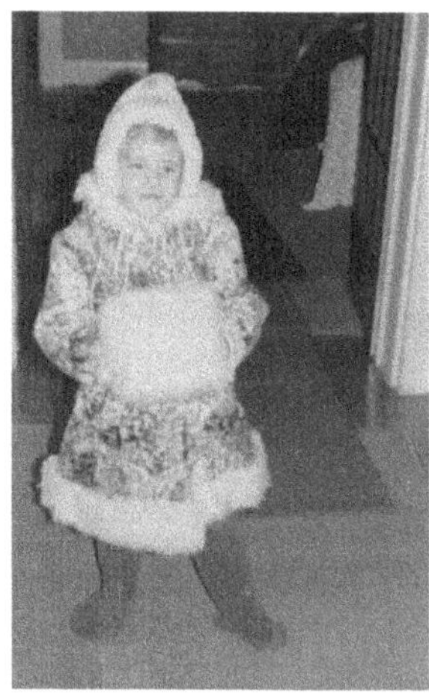

CHILDHOOD

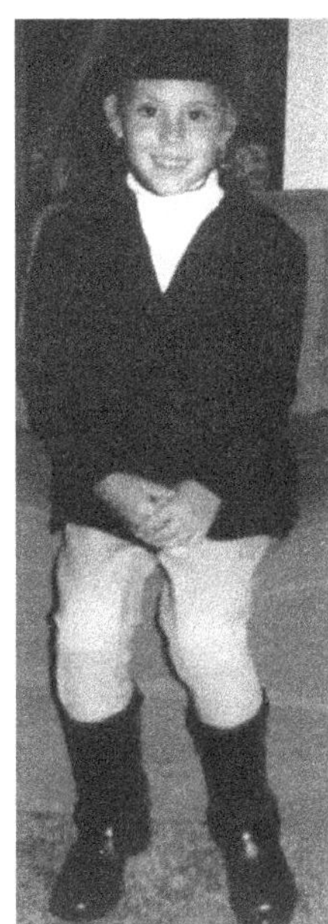
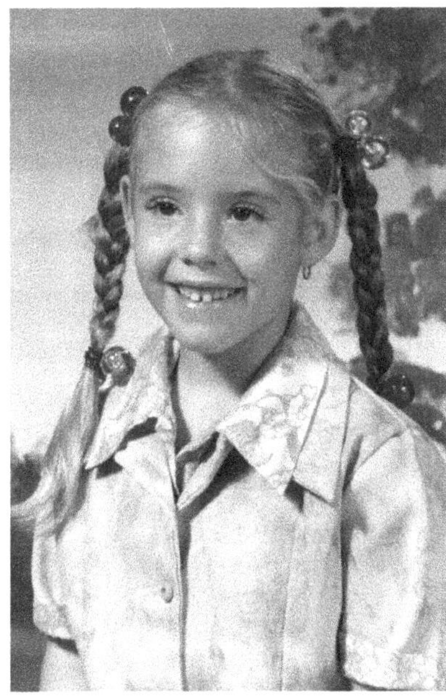
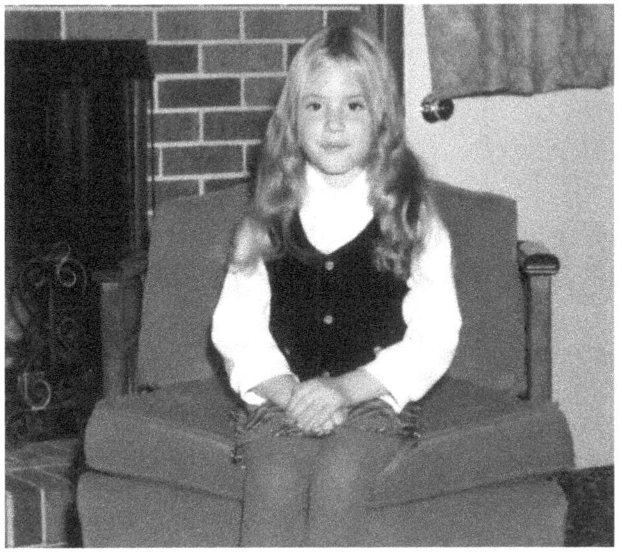

COLLEGE

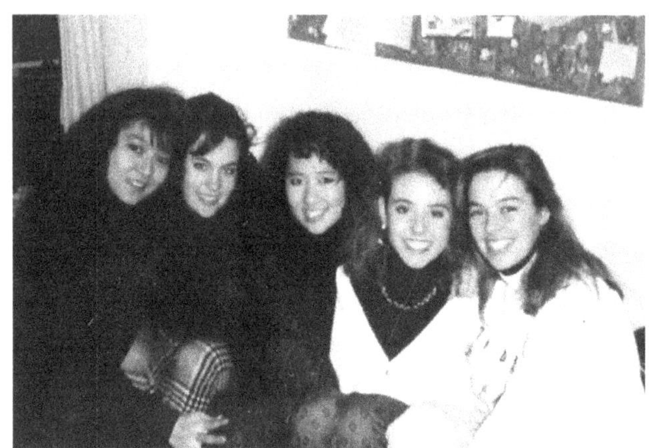

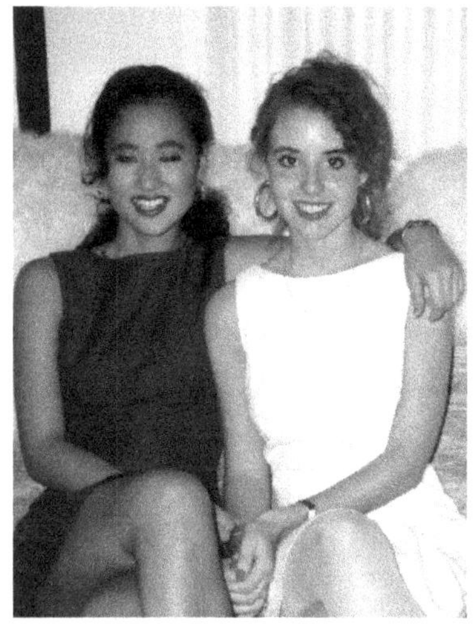

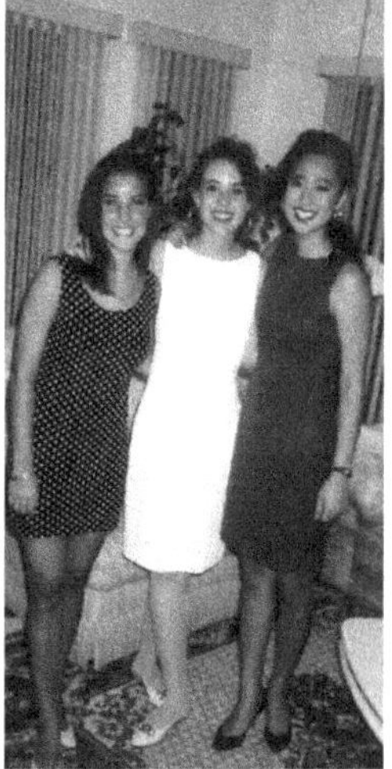

COLLEGE

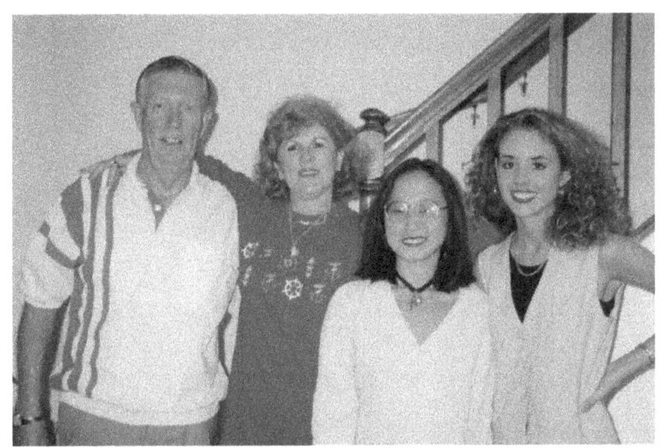

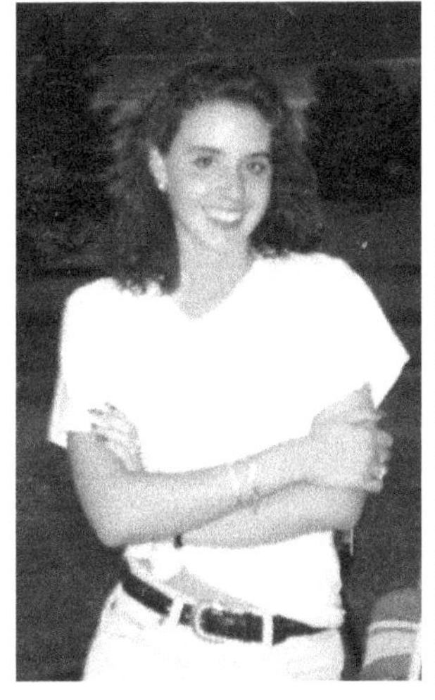

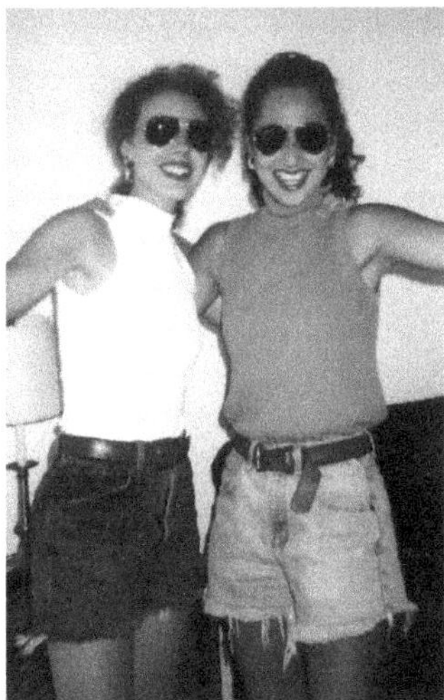

WEDDING DAY

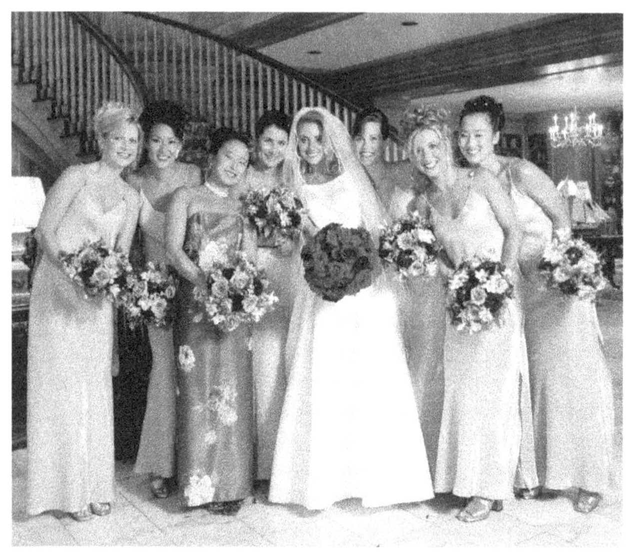

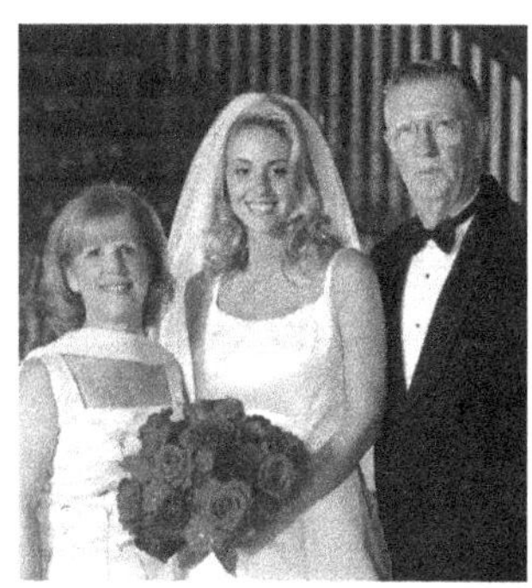

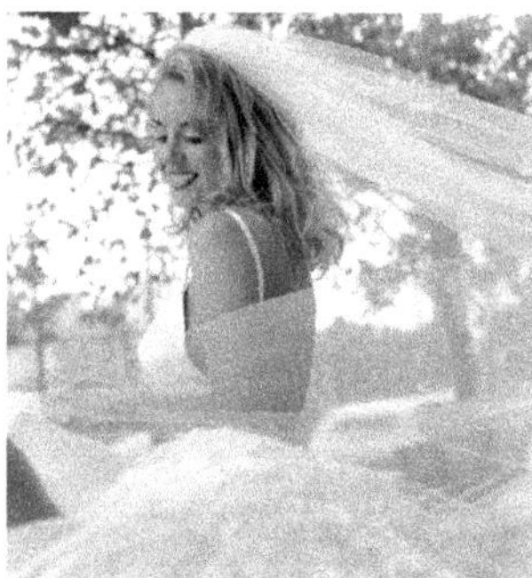

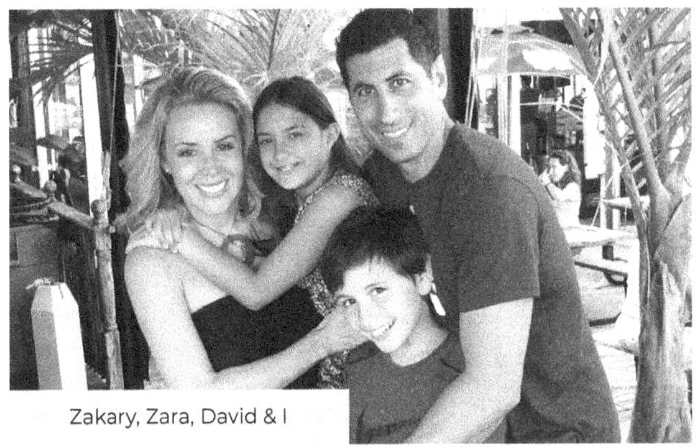

Zakary, Zara, David & I

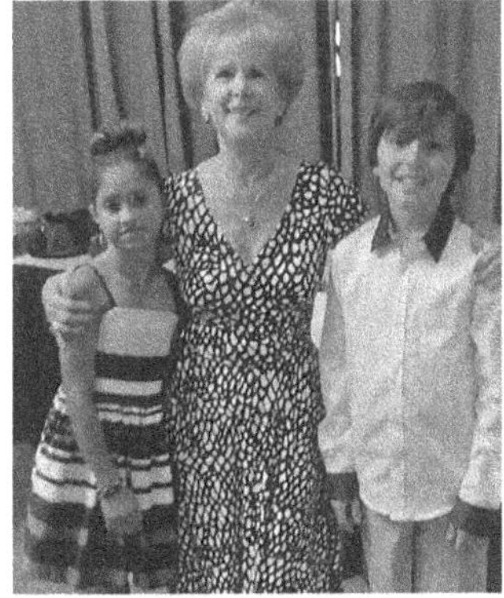

My mother, Zakary & Zara

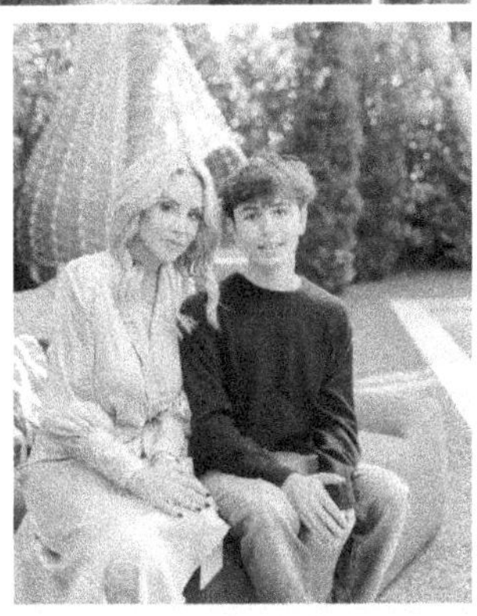

My son Zakary & I

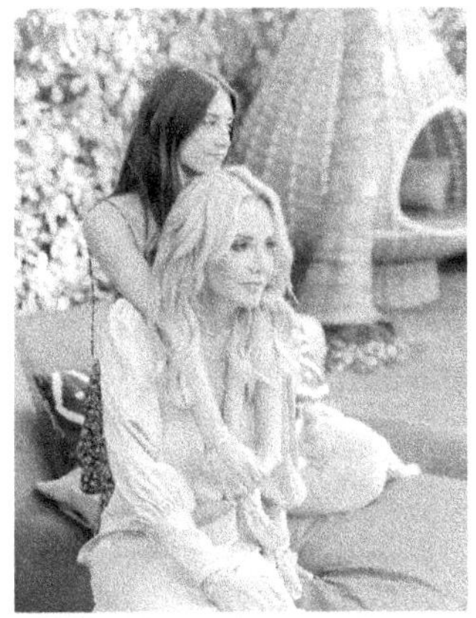

My daughter Zara & I

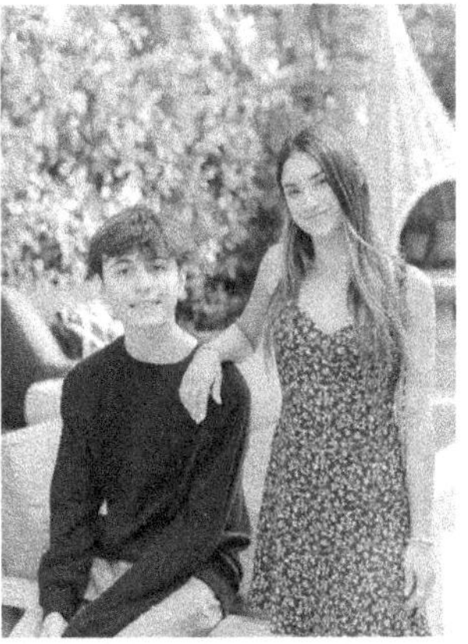

Zakary & Zara

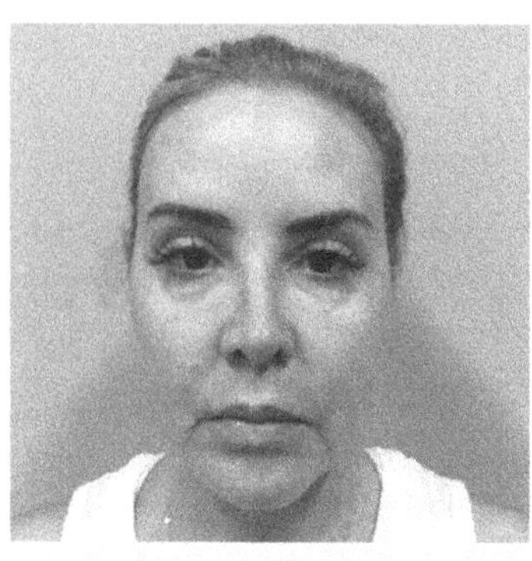

Before face lift picture

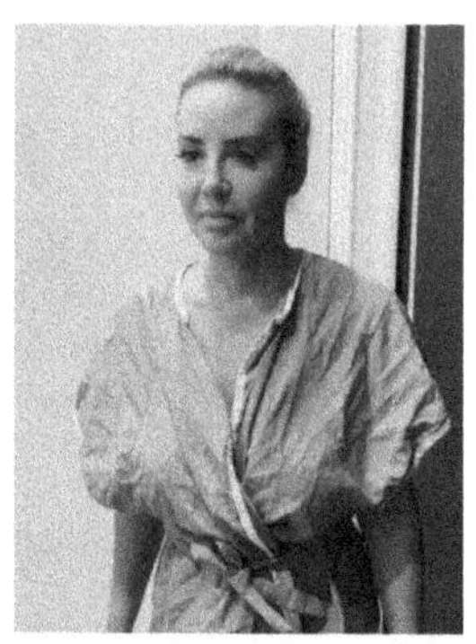

Going into my face lift

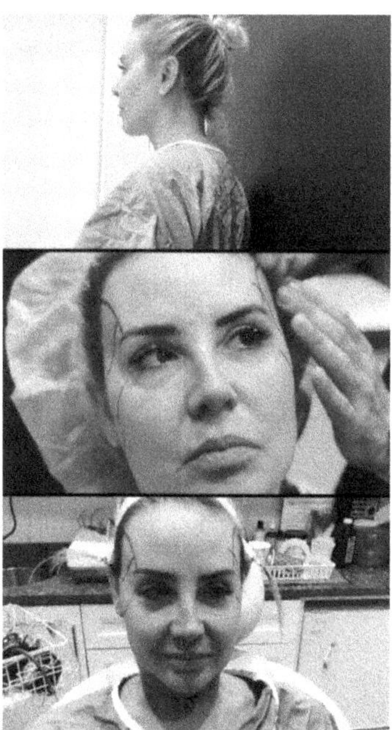

Dr. Jacono marking up my face
prior to the face lift

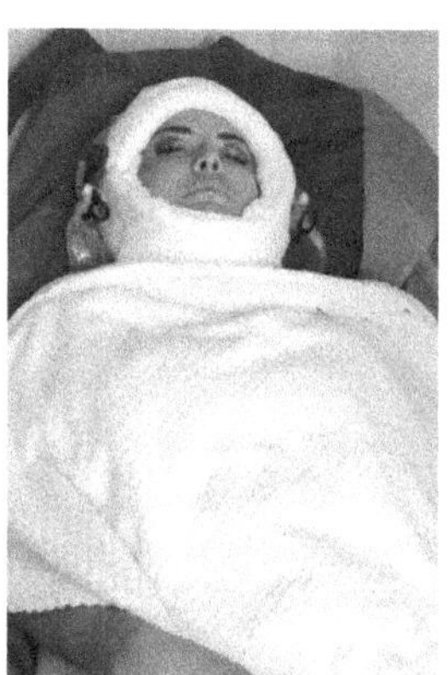

Right after my face lift

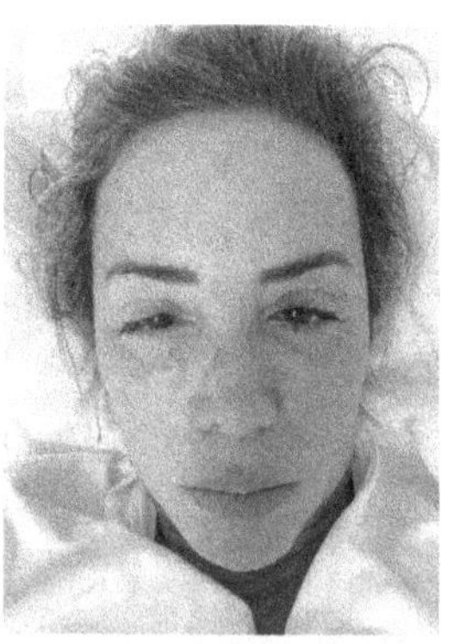

Dengue fever

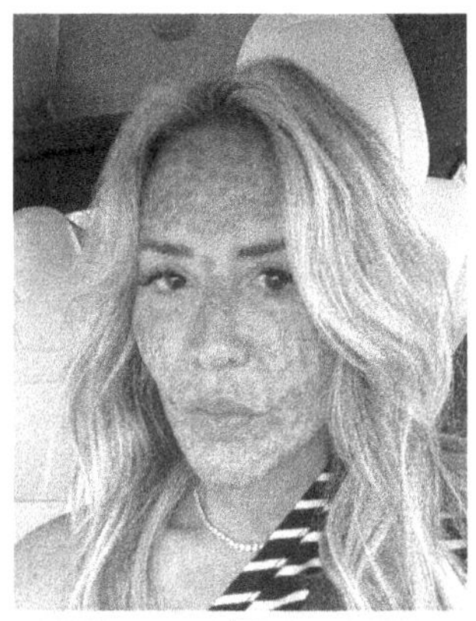

Co2 Selfie!

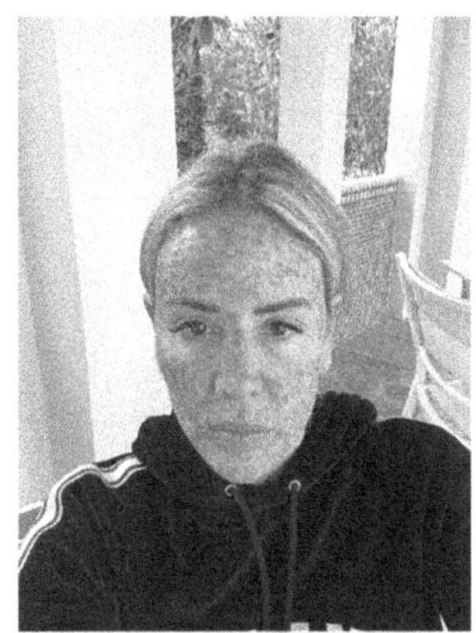

CO2 laser

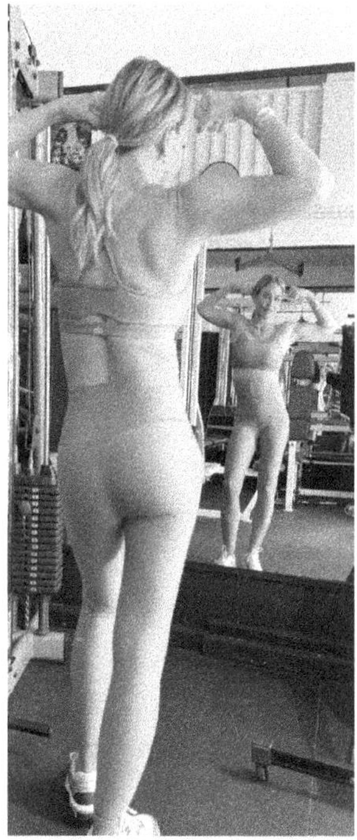

Working out at Hiperfit with
my trainer Vanessa

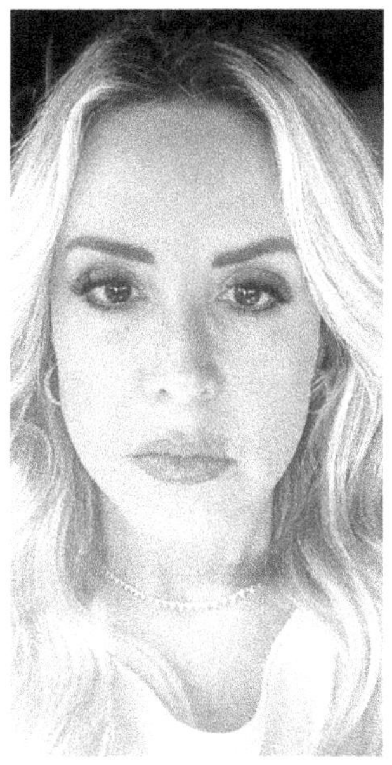

After face lift picture

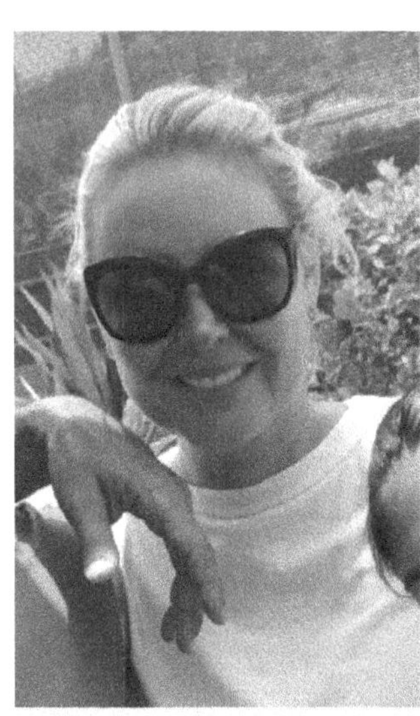

Face swollen before
lymphatic drainage

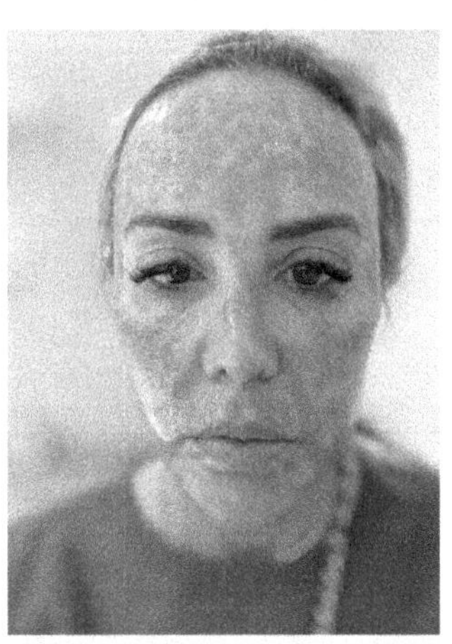

CO2 laser

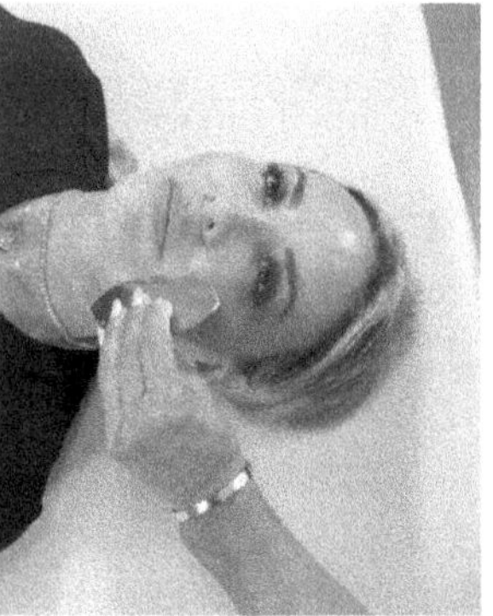

Face gua sha work
with Vanessa

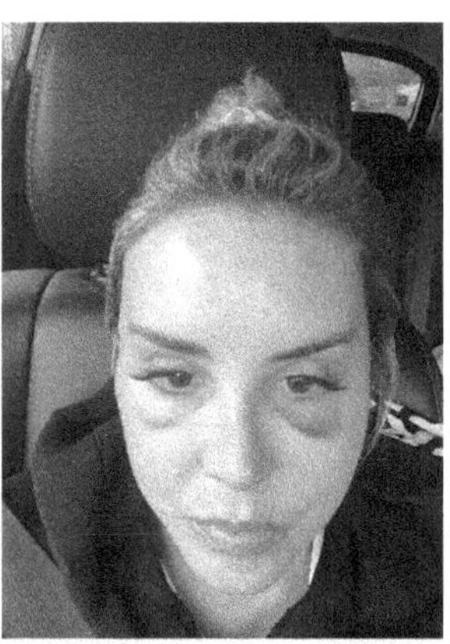

After my face lift healing

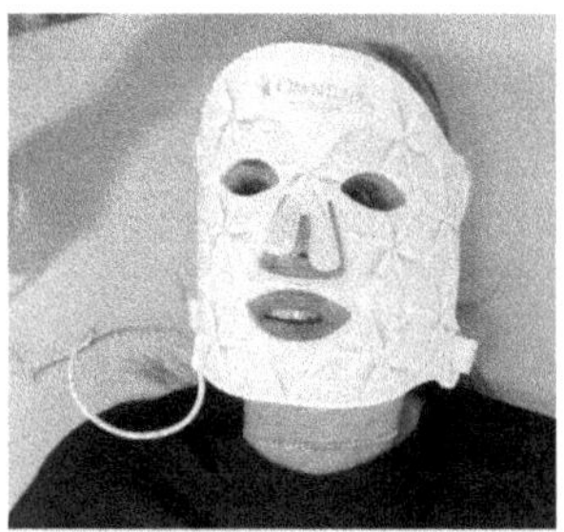

Omnilux red light therapy

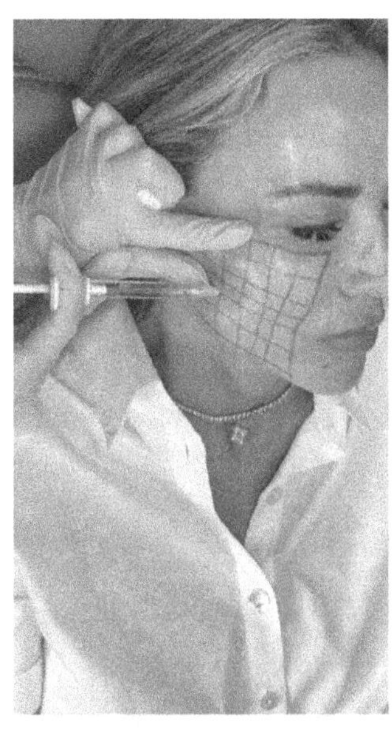

Skinvive treatment

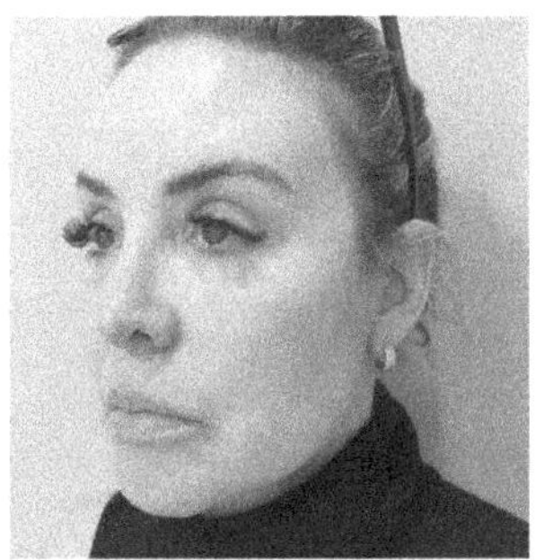

Before face lift-
face was swollen

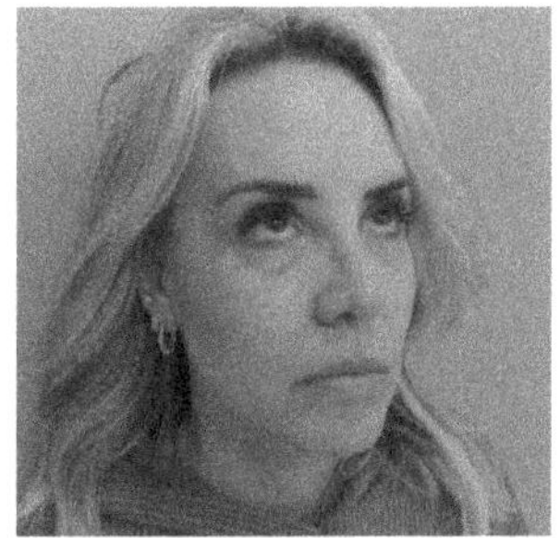

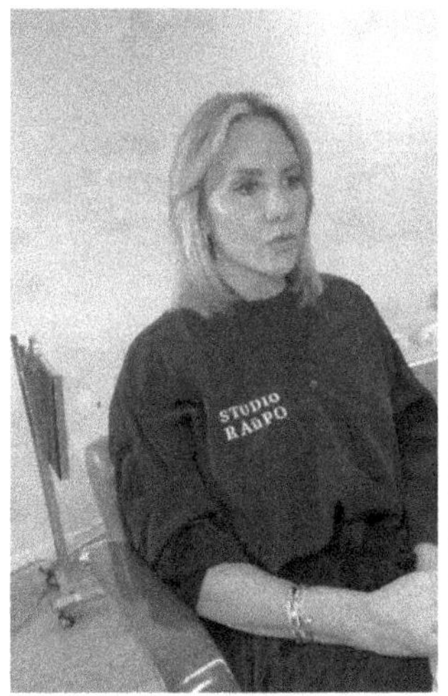

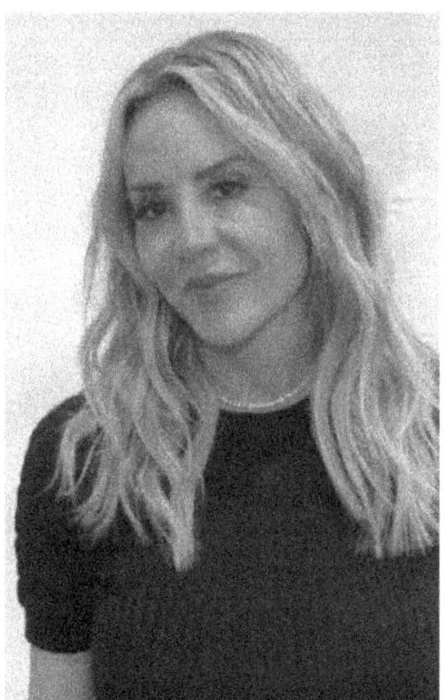

Hair extensions before and after!

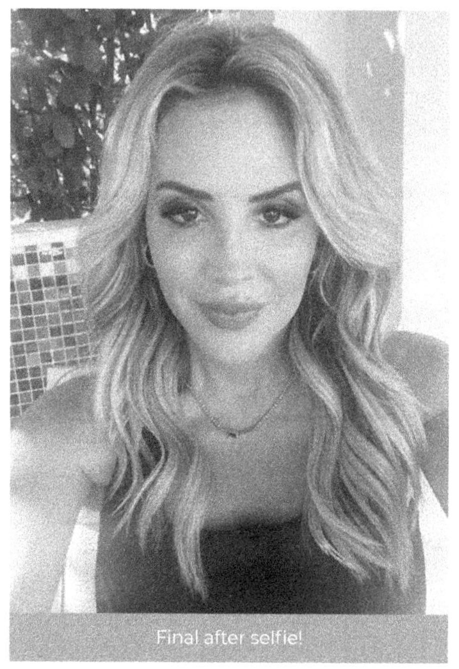
Final after selfie!

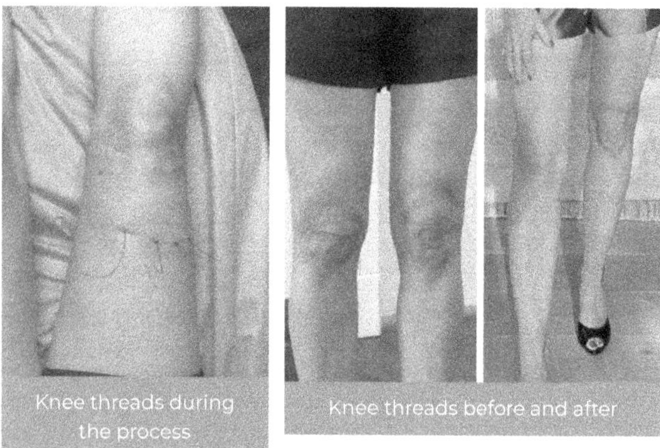
Knee threads during the process

Knee threads before and after

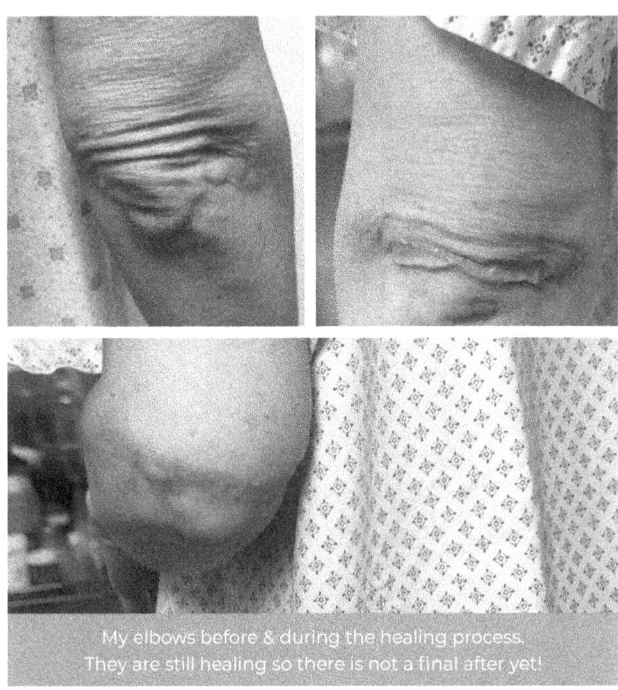

My elbows before & during the healing process.
They are still healing so there is not a final after yet!

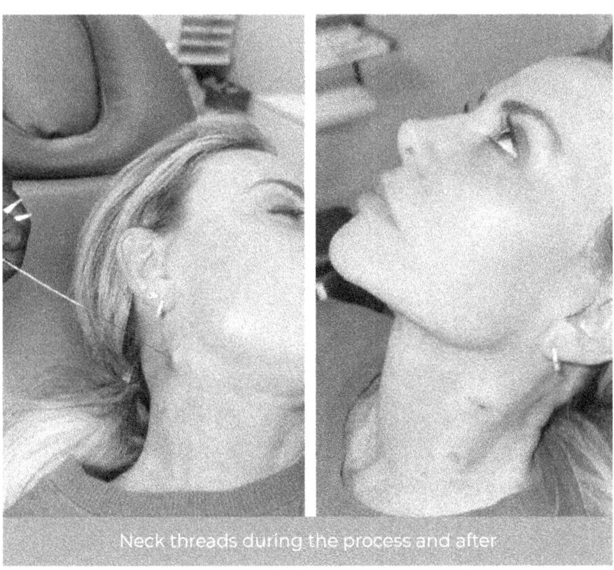

Neck threads during the process and after

PHOTOSHOOT WITH ANDRES OYUELA

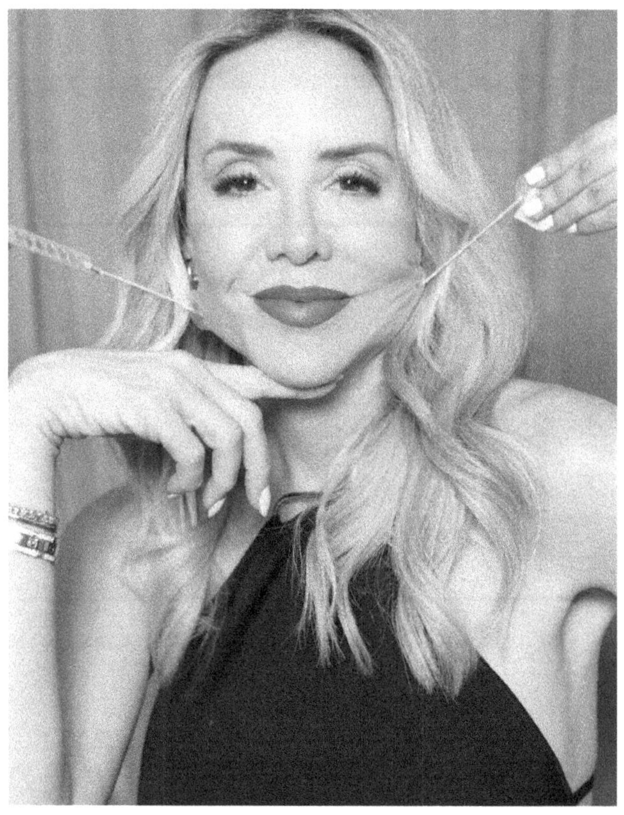

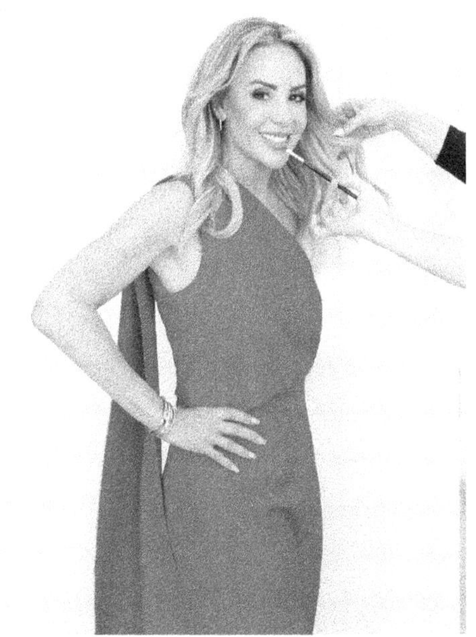

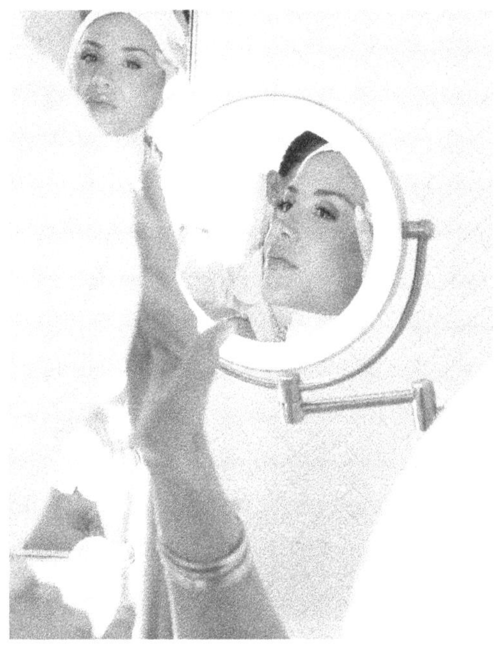

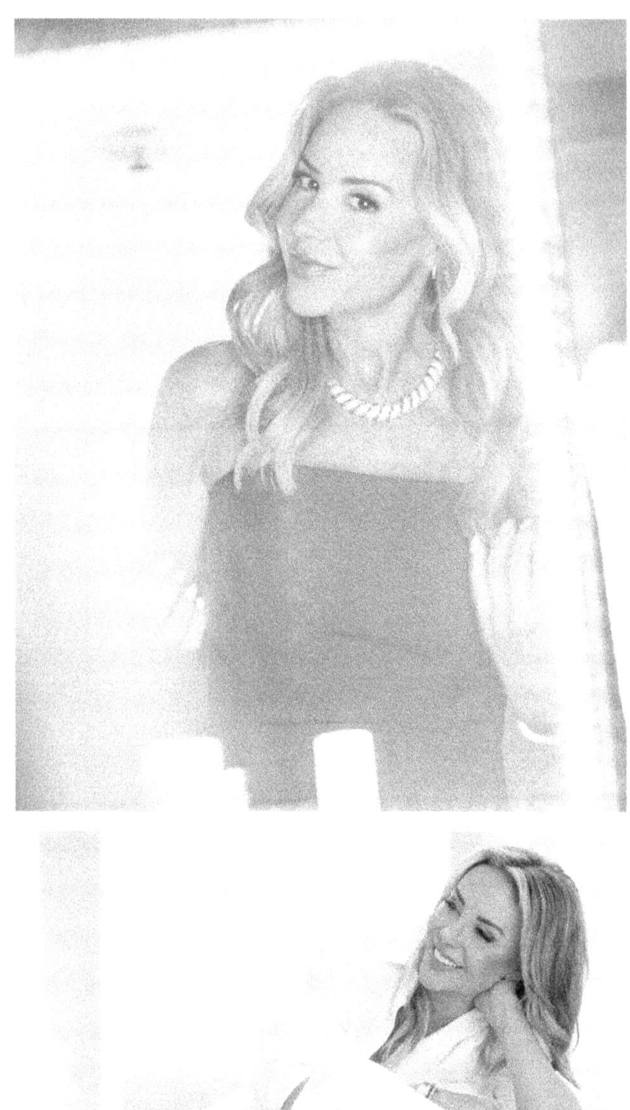

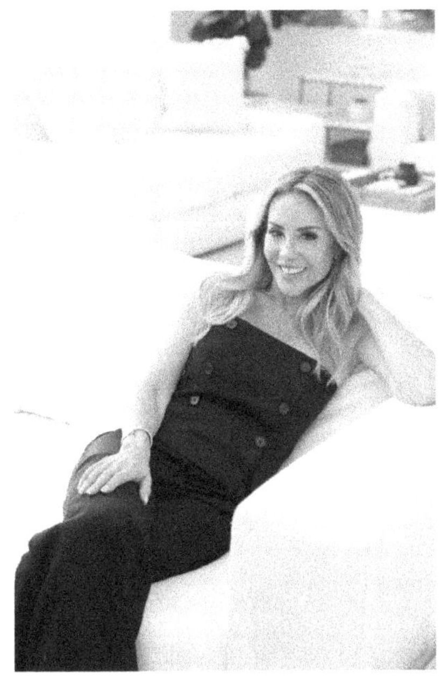

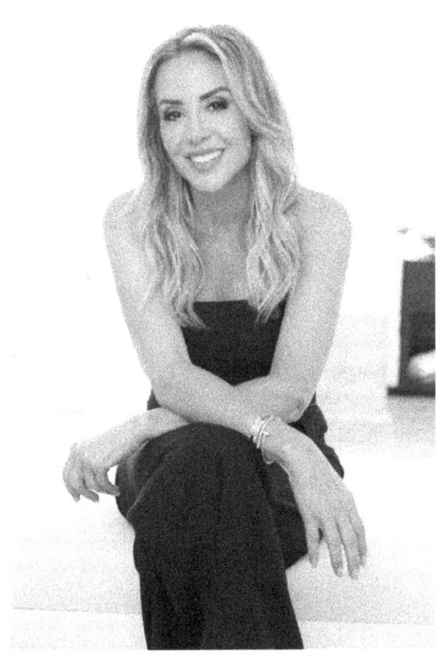

Must-Nose About Rhinoplasty

Now let's discuss a surgery topic that wasn't so much of a love-at-first-sight story for me as it was a slow burn. And that's rhinoplasties.

A rhinoplasty is the surgical term for a nose job. I got my first rhinoplasty in my twenties and it was honestly underwhelming. I went to a doctor in Baltimore and received his signature style: these itty-bitty noses. During our consultation, I described what I wanted, that is a *normal* size nose, not a teeny tiny one. I trusted he would listen and not take his typical approach with me. I was wrong—UGH! I left his office with a nose that was just...*too small.* I didn't like it. While it was better than what I had started out with, it wasn't what I wanted, and I kicked myself for not going to someone else. The shape of my nose bothered me for years.

A little while down the road, in a scene reminiscent of that iconic *Brady Bunch* TV episode ("The Subject Was Noses"), someone threw a football and it accidentally hit me in the nose, breaking it. Yes, the situation kind of sucked, but it was also a good excuse to upgrade that little button nose I had been living with. I was weirdly relieved.

This go-round, I went to a different doctor for the rhinoplasty and, though it went better, my nose was still not perfect. I waited a few more years, then repeated the surgery for the last time with a doctor I really liked in Washington, D.C. Finally, I was happy with the outcome! Now, my nose isn't *perfect*, but it's fine. It's not enough for me to go in for another surgery.

So, yes, I've had three rhinoplasties. But I guarantee that there are lots of other women (and women in your own circle, I promise you) who have had at least one! These surgeries are very common today, and many plastic surgeons have perfected their technique to make the results look very natural. Although it took a few tries for me to get something I'm happy with, I'd definitely recommend it to anyone who wants one. Even the subtlest of tweaks to your nose can make a world of a difference when it comes to evening out your face. (They say the world's most beautiful people have perfectly asymmetrical faces…and now you can, too!)

Now, let me break it all down for you. A rhinoplasty is a procedure to enhance the appearance and functionality of the nose. So, some people will get them for aesthetic reasons, while others need the surgery to address breathing issues. (If you've ever heard someone say they have a deviated septum, that's what they're talking about.) I hope this goes without saying, but this procedure should *only* be done by a board-certified plastic surgeon with experience in rhinoplasty. DO NOT TAKE ANY SHORTCUTS TO SAVE MONEY!

Do your research, as always, and be sure to tell your surgeon exactly what you're looking for during your consultation. You don't want any surprises! If and when too much cartilage is removed, you may need a repeat procedure and they'll have to use cartilage from a cadaver. (Back in the day, they used to have to take it from your own rib! Not fun.)

You'll have a consultation first so that you and the surgeon can get clear on your goals and set realistic expectations. The surgeon will also fill you in on what to expect during and after the procedure.

Fortunately, you'll be under anesthesia during a nose job (thank God!!). The surgeon will make incisions to get to the bone of your nose. Then, to put it bluntly, the surgeon will chisel away (sorry, but that's exactly what happens—gah!) to reshape the bone and cartilage for the desired nose structure. The surgery usually takes between one to three hours. When it's over, the recovery can be uncomfortable. I remember being in pain for a few days; there was a lot of swelling and bruising, but nothing some ice, pain meds, and Arnica couldn't help. I laid low for a few days following the surgery and, within a week, I was back to feeling like myself again.

Definitely follow up with your surgeon so that the doctor can monitor your healing, address any of your concerns, remove splints or stitches, and make any needed adjustments. Be aware that sometimes it can take up to several months to see the full results due to ongoing swelling. So be patient if you don't see the exact results you want right out of the gate.

As with facelifts, there are similar risks when getting a nose job: excessive bleeding, infection, anesthesia complications, scarring, asymmetry, and breathing difficulties. There's also the risk that you won't love the results (just like with mine). But getting the right surgeon is the best way to avoid these risks.

Expect to pay between $5,000 and $15,000 for a rhinoplasty. Sometimes insurance will help with the cost if there's a medical reason for the surgery. However, if the intention is purely for cosmetic purposes, you might be out of luck. Definitely ask about payment plan options; just like with facelifts, it's an option that can be really helpful.

Facelifts and rhinoplasties are both so common today that there's really no reason to fear going under the knife for them. If you want a nose job, and can afford it, don't let anything stop you! While both facelifts and rhinoplasties carry their own considerations and potential risks, each can lead to a huge improvement in your confidence (and appearance). Let me be your surgical cheerleader: Go for it!

CHAPTER SIX

HOT GIRL BODY 101

Oh, to be thin! To have great boobs! To be tight *downtown!* Arguably, there isn't a woman on the planet who doesn't want at least one of these, especially those of us who are aging. We all want a hot girl body! And sometimes that requires a bit of surgical help. Let me teach you the ways…

First, we have that stubborn fat! Women have been told for… well, FOREVER, that we need to be thin to be considered beautiful. So, we've done everything to achieve it. Every fad diet: Atkins, Keto, South Beach, Paleo, Whole30, the freakin' grapefruit diet! Every exercise program and device, including Zumba, Jazzercise, vibrating belts, and the ThighMaster.

And when all else fails, we've reduced some of that stubborn fat through surgery and procedures like liposuction and body sculpting. We've pulled out all of the stops to feel confident and comfortable in our bodies. The surgical means to this end are helpful, even if they are only temporary fixes. Let's get right into the basics of these procedures, their benefits, and everything else you need to know if you're looking to get fat sucked out or moved around.

The Real Skinny on Lipo

Is liposuction worth it? For me, the answer to this has been mixed.

But let's start with what it is, for anyone who's been living under a rock. Liposuction is one of the most well-known types of plastic surgery. It's been around since 1975, and for some people, it's been phenomenal. Liposuction is a procedure that literally sucks the fat out of areas of the body, anywhere you think you might have too much. During the brief procedure, a plastic surgeon will use a suction device to remove the fat deposits through small incisions made in the body. Today, doctors use it to remove excess fat deposits from the butt, thighs, stomach, and even underarms. It's not a weight-loss technique, but more of a body contouring method that naturally enhances what God gave you. (So, if you have more than 100 pounds of weight to lose, this is not a viable option to achieve that goal).

The first time I tried liposuction was in my thirties, right after I had my son, Zakary. That particular experience went great, and I was really happy with the results. It was technically liposuction, but the technology wasn't what it is today, so it seemed like the fat was *repositioned* more than removed—I'd consider it more of a sculpting technique.

It was done using a small wand that basically melted the fat and distributed it to other parts of the body. It was a six-and-a-half-hour procedure—starting with the arms and working down, melting and sculpting along the way. (I especially loved what the doctor did with my inner thighs because it gave me a diamond shaped look there.) Overall, I looked a lot smaller after, but it did involve some work on my end too. After the procedure, I had to wear this tight garment under my clothes every day for two months. I also had to get medical massages every week during that time. I followed the doctor's instructions exactly, though, and while it wasn't a weight loss technique, I did lose inches (I went from a size 27 in jeans to a size 25). I loved the way I looked.

Then, I tried liposuction again in my early forties, and immediately wished I hadn't. Now, rewind a second back to my botched Y Lift when I'd found a woman in Miami to start removing that terrible face filler. While she was helpful with the filler removal, she caused all sorts of other problems. She happened to perform liposuction at her office, so I figured this was my opportunity to bid farewell to some of that stubborn belly fat. During the liposuction procedure, I was awake the whole time (typically they put you under, so this really *sucked!*) and it hurt so bad. Not to mention, the results were bad too. I had so much saggy skin on my stomach after the surgery that I ended up having to get a mini tummy tuck (which I never needed before).

The lipo doctor also told me that she could liposuction my knees. In the moment, it seemed like a good idea (this was before I'd realized the terrible results on my stomach). Oh, if only I could go back in time! She ended up taking out *too much* fat from my knees, which made them very uneven. Now, with so much fat gone, the skin on my knees started to sag majorly; I had to get threads in them. This is when I also started to get filler in my knees too. I had to go back for tweaks about every five months. All in all, my liposuction experience was terrible.

To make matters worse, I found out that this woman changed her prices for procedures depending on the person. For example, if she thought you had money, she would charge you more. It was all really shady. I've since come to realize that working out over time—specifically weight training—is the best fix to fight fat. (I've built a lot of muscle from following a strict routine, but more on that in a later chapter).

I realized a huge part of why this procedure didn't go well for me is because I went to someone who was not qualified enough to do it. I think if I had found the right doctor, it would have been a far better experience. Let's talk about the ideal patient and what the process normally looks like.

1. The ideal patient for liposuction is someone with localized areas of excess fat that are resistant to diet and exercise. You know what I mean…those pockets of fat that never seem to go away. Common areas include the stomach, thighs, hips, butt, arms, chin, and neck.

2. Liposuction is best for people who are close to their ideal weight. It's also best for someone with good skin elasticity, as this prevents too much saggy skin. (Also keep in mind that, while liposuction can suck out the unwanted fat, it does not take care of the loose skin that will be left behind. This is something else to consider and talk about with your doctor.)

3. The patient is put under anesthesia. Then the surgeon will make small incisions near the targeted areas.

4. The surgeon inserts a cannula to loosen excess fat deposits. A suction device is then attached to the cannula to remove the fat cells, contouring the body to the desired shape.

5. The recovery time is pretty quick. Most patients can resume normal activities within a few days. Doctors recommend wearing compression clothing during the recovery period to reduce swelling and support the healing process. While there is some extent of pain, it's nothing pain medication can't manage.

Risks for liposuction include bleeding, infection, fluid buildup, changes in skin sensation, contour irregularities, and scarring. Ultimately though, if it's done right, you can leave looking more sculpted and better than ever. And for the cost (usually about $6,000 per treatment area), it can be well worth it.

Just as with any of these treatments, it's important to be realistic about the results. Again, if you have tons of fat to lose, it's better to get a head start with the right diet and exercise, if you're not already doing so.

Other Body Sculpting & Contouring Techniques

Now on to sculpting and contouring techniques. So, while liposuction procedures these days focus primarily on fat removal, body sculpting techniques include skin tightening, muscle toning, or fat grafting for more comprehensive results. Here are some popular types of sculpting and contouring out there these days. I'm sure you've heard of a lot of these:

Tummy Tucks

The tummy tuck, which is surgically called an abdominoplasty, is a very popular procedure; however, it is far more intense than liposuction. It focuses on toning, flattening, and tightening any loose skin on the stomach. As I mentioned, I had a mini tummy tuck in my forties after my second liposuction experience went terribly and left behind all that saggy skin.

During a tummy tuck, the patient will be under anesthesia. The surgeon then makes an incision across the lower abdomen to remove excess skin and fat and tighten the abdominal muscles. The remaining skin is then repositioned for a smoother, firmer contour of the stomach. Speaking from experience, I didn't find this to be painful and my recovery was fine. (It was a bit uncomfortable with swelling, bruising, and soreness, but overall, nothing crazy.) I was able to easily get rid of the scar with laser treatments.

Risks for a tummy tuck are similar to other surgeries and include infection, excess bleeding, scarring, and complications related to anesthesia. A tummy tuck usually costs between $5,000 and $15,000.

(Oh! And I'm sure you've heard of the "mommy makeover." That's a combination of liposuction, a tummy tuck, and a breast enhancement to help with post-pregnancy body changes. It's all very customizable. I know plenty of moms who've done this after having children, and the changes in their appearance—and their self-esteem—are remarkable. Costs vary greatly depending on the customization, but expect to pay upward of $20,000.)

If you choose to try these options, keep in mind that you need to maintain a healthy lifestyle to get the most time out of the procedures. Nothing lasts forever, but you can at least maintain these treatments for a while if you're good to your body. Diet and exercise are so, so important. (Stay with me to the end of the book for much more on this!)

CoolSculpting & SculpSure

Personally, I hate these procedures and don't find them helpful at all, but I want to talk about them anyway. You might have a totally different experience.

CoolSculpting is a non-invasive procedure that—just like liposuction—targets fat deposits. But instead of sucking the fat out, it freezes, then destroys, fat cells. During the procedure, the CoolSculpting device is applied to the target area of fat, where it delivers controlled cooling to freeze the fat cells without damaging surrounding tissues. Over several weeks, the body naturally eliminates the destroyed fat cells, resulting in gradual fat reduction and improved body contours.

Sounds good in theory…but I've never noticed any results from this. And I don't know anyone who has. But, let's carry on.

CoolSculpting isn't painful; the device feels like it pulls and tugs your body and it's definitely *cold.* The process only takes about thirty to sixty minutes for each treatment area. Potential risks are limited to temporary numbness, redness, swelling, bruising, and skin sensitivity at the treatment site.

As with lipo, CoolSculpting definitely isn't the right fit for someone who has a lot of weight to lose. The cost ranges between $2,000 and $4,000 per session. I'll say explore this at your own risk— the risk of wasting money!

SculpSure is a concept similar to CoolSculpting, but instead of freezing the fat, SculpSure uses a laser to heat and destroy the fat cells. Again, this is targeted, so the focus areas tend to be the stomach, love handles, thighs, and under the chin. The sessions are shorter than CoolSculpting and usually take about twenty-five minutes. There is no pain and rarely any discomfort either—maybe a warmth or tingling in the targeted areas, but that's it.

Again, I found zero success with this, but plenty of people out there like it. Usually results (for people who see them) start to show up within a few weeks. Cost per session tends to range between $1,500 and $3,000, so it's very similar to CoolSculpting in that regard too.

I've had both procedures, and I don't think they work—and they're *not* worth the money, or time. I like to see quick results as well, and both of these procedures take a while to show those results. (This is why I get filler in the spots where cellulite shows up. Then I have instantaneous results.)

Brazilian Butt Lift
(Better Known as a "BBL")

Something that's been very trendy in recent years is the Brazilian Butt Lift or BBL. (Fun fact: It's called the Brazilian Butt Lift because the surgery was pioneered by Ivo Pitanguy—a surgeon from Brazil.) It gives women who don't have much back *there* something to work with. It's for my flat-booty-ed ladies who want to enhance those curves with a shapely butt.

Now, I have a naturally bountiful booty, so I've never considered this type of fat transferal, but I'll still tell you a little about it. The procedure starts with liposuction of fat from one area of the patient's body. The fat is then purified and injected into the butt. It's sort of like a two-for-one deal: The person removes fat from an unwanted spot on their body and builds up fat in the area they *do* want it. Using a person's own body fat helps avoid the rare complications associated with implants, which can include infection, capsular contracture (scar tissue tightening around the implant), implant rupture or leakage, implant displacement, and allergic reactions.

Once the procedure is complete, there is minimal scarring, and the recovery time is short. If done by the right surgeon, the results can look great and natural. But like with anything else, the wrong doctor can leave you botched. I've heard absolute horror stories about women coming to Miami to meet with shady doctors for this procedure on a dime and ending up dead—DEAD! (If the deal on the BBL seems *too good*, it is!) Is it truly worth risking your life for a fatter booty? I'd vote no.

How can a poorly done BBL lead to death? Here's how: It can cause a fat embolism, where the injected fat accidentally enters the bloodstream and blocks blood vessels. This can then lead to respiratory or cardiac arrest.

Listen, I don't think there's anything wrong with getting a BBL so long as you go to the right professional to do it—someone who is board certified and truly an expert. I know some people who've gotten a BBL, and their results didn't seem to last long, which is weird. I've heard a BBL can last up to decades, but I haven't personally witnessed this. Experts in the field say that once the transferred fat establishes a blood supply in its new location in the body, it will become permanent and that results can last many years. Again, I just don't see it. And the cost? Expect to pay between $4,000 and $10,000 for a BBL.

This is my honest take. Yes, BBLs have risen in popularity, but times are changing! If you're looking to make your booty more *booty-ful,* you'll achieve longer effects through weight training (which also helps get rid of cellulite, too, but we'll get to that later) and it will look more natural too. Nothing is better than putting in the work when it comes to the butt. It took my personal trainer, Vanessa, ten years to build her butt naturally through diet and exercise, but she's a great example of how it *can* be done!

Fat Transfer

The butt isn't the only place with a welcome mat for fat transfers. Fat transferal is also popular in the face and breasts (common injection sites).

The face: The idea is to fill in any hollow-looking areas, like under the eyes or the cheeks, to give the face an overall younger appearance.

The breasts: With breast augmentation, the fat injections can enhance the volume and shape of the breasts without implants. (Women tend to like this for a natural and subtle look.)

As with the BBL, the procedure removes fat from one area of the body (where it's unwanted). The fat is then purified and injected into the target area. This can be a good alternative to implants and fillers, but again, talk to a board-certified doctor about the best option for you. Fat transfer isn't for everyone, and many different factors can contribute to whether you're even a candidate or not, including your weight, skin elasticity, goals, and overall health.

Depending upon the area the body fat is being transferred to and from, you can expect to pay between $2,500 and $7,000. Results (for those who experience them) are usually seen in about six months.

Kybella

Kybella (which is technically an injectable) is commonly used to reduce fat under the chin—the dreaded "double chin." I consider myself lucky that I've never had fat build up under my chin, but plenty of women (and men) do and they want it *gone*. So, it's become pretty popular.

But a lot of people don't realize that Kybella can be used on other fat pockets on the body too. My injector, Denise Santoli did Kybella for me on a banana roll I had under my butt, and it worked like a charm. She's told me Kybella works for small pockets of stubborn fat, like the banana rolls, as well as love handles, muffin tops, buccal fat, inner thighs, and knee fat. If you're on the heavier side and are looking to get rid of a lot of fat in a rather big area, Kybella isn't going to be the best option. Also, people who tend to have the best results with this have good skin elasticity, like with other treatments.

The Kybella injections contain synthetic deoxycholic acid, which is a naturally occurring molecule in the body that helps the breakdown and absorption of dietary fat. You can get Kybella treatments from an injector like I did, so a surgeon isn't required; I'd still recommend that if you want the procedure to find someone who is well-trained in this injectable and whose patients have experienced good results with it.

Kybella is injected directly into the fat, and it only takes about fifteen to twenty minutes. For the first week after I got Kybella, the injection area swelled up to about three times the size, but Denise assured me this was normal. The swelling slowly got better, and the full extent of the results showed up in about a month. My banana roll was gone!

Most patients have to come back for a series of treatments, which are spaced around four to six weeks apart. Each treatment can usually cost upwards of $600. If you can't stand your double chin and don't want surgery or lipo, this can definitely be an option for you.

As I'm sure you've gathered by now, I don't *fully love* any of these fat removal or fat transferal procedures, but they can be helpful, depending. Again, to each their own! If any of them sound interesting to you, seek out the right doctor and do a consultation beforehand.

Enhancing the Ladies

My boobs were the first thing I ever got done. I was in my twenties and I was tired of my *blah* A-cup. I went to a doctor in Baltimore who totally overdid it with the implants. I left with a size that looked and felt uncomfortably large for my smaller frame.

On the positive side, my bounce-back time was only a couple of days and there wasn't a whole ton of pain like I'd expected. I was back at work within a few days. (The doctor had advised me not to work out for a month, but I didn't listen. I did some light lifting focusing on my legs and abs, and I was totally fine).

In the years following the birth of my son, Zakary, my body no longer looked how I wanted it to. There was so much scar tissue built up in my boobs that they looked bigger than ever, and I hated that unnatural look so much. So, in my forties I decided to get a replacement implant—something significantly smaller and better suited for my body type—and a breast lift with Dr. Michelle Zweifler in New York City (www.drmichellezweifler.com). I figured in the two decades since my previous experience, advancements in these surgeries would mean a far better result, and I was right. (Not to mention Dr. Zweifler is AMAZING!)

During my surgery with Dr. Zweifler, she removed the original implants (and got rid of that scar tissue), replacing them with smaller implants. She also removed any loose skin and gave my boobs a lift. I now have a smaller size that looks so much better on me. Plus, there is nothing better than having perky ladies in my fifties! I never shy away from wearing a bathing suit because I'm confident as could be!

Sizing Up with Breast Implants

Women get breast implants because they want bigger boobs, more volume and/or an improved shape. (Here's where you're thinking, "Thank you Captain Obvious!") Implants are medical devices (it seems weird to think of them as *devices*, but it's technically what they are) that are inserted into the chest. There are two types that are most typically used—silicone gel implants and saline implants. Both implant types have a silicone outer layer, but the former are filled with silicone gel, and the latter are filled with sterile saltwater. Silicone implants tend to give a more natural look and feel, and they come in a wide range of shapes and sizes depending on what you're looking for. Saline implants have a firmer feel and are adjustable during and after surgery, meaning you can slightly increase or decrease the size. Both types of devices are monitored for leaks by your doctor (but in today's world, leaks are less likely).

I have a narrow frame, which means I needed a high-profile breast. A low or moderate profile is great for women with a wider build. This is why it's so important to talk to your doctor to make sure you're getting the right implant device for your profile. (If you've ever seen one of those ladies whose fake boobs look big enough to topple them over, they have the wrong profile!)

Breast implants can be a total game changer! Any great board-certified surgeon will engage in a thorough consultation with you to discuss your goals, medical history, and the different options available. Together, you'll figure out the right implant shape and size and the best placement for your body and profile. Dr. Zweifler would certainly agree that this entire process *needs* to be personalized to you.

On the day of my procedure, I went in ready to go under. Usually, the procedure takes between one and three hours. Mine was on the lengthier side, mostly because we did the implant removal and lift too. I was nervous about scarring afterward, but thanks to some laser treatments later, I have no scarring at all. I was prescribed pain medication, which I took for a few days, and I took it easy during that stretch of time, but overall, the downtime was not bad. Longer term, I avoided any heavy lifting for a few weeks to make sure I had the best results.

I've said it before and I'll say it again: Nothing in the world of plastic surgery is permanent, and this applies to breast implants too. They're not guaranteed to last a lifetime and, depending on when you get them, you may need to have them replaced or removed over time. If you do decide to get implants, be sure to check in with your surgeon for regular follow-up appointments to monitor them. This will help you stay ahead of any possible concerns too.

I couldn't recommend breast implants more for anyone who's considering them. Whether you're rocking a bikini at the beach or wearing your favorite little black dress with a plunging neckline, your enhanced curves can bring you a ton of confidence. On average, you can expect breast implants to cost somewhere between $5,000 and $19,000, depending on factors like your location and the doctor.

Now, let's hear Dr. Zweifler's take on the topic of breast implants.

BREAST IMPLANTS
Words from the Wise:
Michelle Zweifler, M.D.

When it comes to any plastic surgery, it's not just about the surgery, it's also about making sure the patient is mentally and physically prepared for the journey ahead. I spend a lot of time on the consultation with a new client. We talk about everything from their medical history and their recent mammograms to their lifestyle (smoking is one of the worst things my patients can do—and it really negatively impacts their healing time), to anesthesia. Anesthesia is big concern for patients, but we work closely with board-certified anesthesiologists to ensure a safe and comfortable experience. We also talk about the reasons they're doing the surgery, and the skin quality to determine what is the best option for them. Breast implants can also be used to complement a breast lift to help the patient restore volume and fullness.

We can either use saline or silicone implants when doing the procedure. Grafting is another option too, where we take fat from other areas of the patient's body through liposuction, and we inject that into the breasts for volume. The benefit of this is that there's minimal scarring. (This isn't an option for a patient who wants a significant increase in size, though.) There can be concerns with this if it's not done by a very experienced surgeon, though. Always prioritize your safety! Do your research! And be sure to ask your (board-certified) plastic surgeon a lot of questions heading into this.

I tell my patients who are smokers to stop four weeks before surgery. After surgery, patients should not do cardio for three weeks, and no weight lifting for six weeks. They'll also have to wear a bra around the clock for six weeks. After breast implants, it's usually about six months to a year before the scaring begins to lessen.

Perking Up with a Breast Lift

Do you dream of perky, youthful breasts that defy gravity? (Don't we all!) Just like many of us don't love sagging skin elsewhere on our bodies, droopy boobs can make women feel self-conscious too. If your boobs are sagging, a breast lift could be a great option for you. The breast lift procedure lifts and reshapes breasts that have started to droop due to aging, weight changes, pregnancy and breastfeeding, genetics, or other life changes. Whether you're looking to reverse the effects of gravity or simply enhance your natural shape, a breast lift could be your ticket to looking *fine*.

If you're considering a lift, schedule a consultation with a plastic surgeon who specializes in lifts to talk about your goals, concerns, and expectations. The plastic surgeon will assess your breast shape, size, and skin elasticity to determine the best approach for your lift.

The lift surgery can be done in a couple of hours. Just like breast implant surgery, the downtime isn't too bad; you'll have to take it easy for a few days and you'll get some pain medication for any discomfort. Make sure to schedule follow-up appointments with your surgeon to monitor your progress, address any concerns, and help you through the healing process.

BREAST LIFTS
Words from the Wise:
Michelle Zweifler, M.D.

In a standard breast lift, we reposition the breast tissue, remove the excess skin, and sculpt the breasts to achieve a look that's lifted. Like with breast implants, I work with my patients to understand what they're looking to achieve, since everyone's individual wants are different.

There are a few common types of breast lifts:

- **Traditional Lift (Anchor Lift):** This classic lift technique involves creating an anchor-shaped incision around the areola, down the center of the breast, and along the breast crease. It's ideal for significant sagging and provides dramatic results. There will be scarring with the traditional method.

- **Vertical Lift (Lollipop Lift):** With this technique, your surgeon makes a lollipop-shaped incision around the areola and down the breast's center. It's a good option for women with moderate sagging and it results in way less scarring.

- **Peri-Areolar Lift (Donut Lift):** For minor sagging, the peri-areolar lift involves making a vertical incision around the areola. It's the least invasive option and leaves minimal scarring.

On average, a breast lift can run you somewhere between $4,000 and $15,000. Some women will get a breast implant and a breast lift done together (like I did) to get the results they're looking for. Something Dr. Zweifler used during my surgery to help extend how long my breast lift would last was something called breast mesh. It's a synthetic material (don't worry, it's safe for the body) that gives additional support to the breast tissue and to my implants. The breast mesh is customizable, too, and the right surgeon will be able to guide you in that if you're interested and help you decide what's best for you.

Lastly, here's my opinion about timing: If you're considering a breast lift but are planning to get pregnant, definitely wait to get the lift until after you've had kids. Pregnancy will without a doubt impact your breasts, and if you do a lift before, you'll just have to repeat the lift afterward. But if you're done having kids or don't plan on getting pregnant in the future, I say go for it and lift those ladies! The young boobs you've been dreaming of can be yours.

One More Lift to Mention: Elbows

Before we move on, I want to mention another type of lift Dr. Zweifler does at her office that is phenomenal—the elbow lift. Of all the skin on our bodies, our elbow skin is one of the first to show signs of aging. (I've run into celebrities—I need not name names—around my neighborhood who are hugely famous for looking young. And when I've seen their elbows…Oh. My. God. It's like they totally forgot to tend to this very important area! Their faces and elbows simply do not match!) Not to toot my own horn, but my elbows match my face! That's after this procedure with Dr. Zweifler, that is.

For years I had loose skin on my elbows, and it drove me *crazy!* I would constantly focus on the skin there and how bad it looked. I hated my elbows so much! In January 2023 I decided to do the elbow lift and it was one of the best things I've done. It was a pretty quick outpatient procedure—you don't even need to go under for it. Dr. Zweilfer removed the extra skin on both elbows, stitched me up, and I was out the door. There were significant scars from this procedure and I'm using a series of CO2 laser treatments with Amy Koberling to flatten those scars (it's not as intensive to flatten scars when compared to using it on the face). Once those scars are flattened, we're going to use a laser called the Vbeam that's specifically used to reduce redness. The last step is to visit Johanna Hedmann to camouflage the scars. (Camouflaging is amazing for scars, but they need to be flat first and the redness needs to be gone, otherwise it leaves a yellow tone behind.)

I followed a similar path with my tummy tuck scar—just swapping the CO2 laser for the IPL laser—and it looks amazing.

(For my knees, I focus on working out, building muscle and keeping muscle tone, and the threads and filler for now. Similar to the elbow lift, the excess skin on the knees can be cut and tightened, but it's trickier, so a less common procedure.)

ELBOW LIFTS
Words from the Wise:
Michelle Zweifler, M.D.

I know lots of women who've tried filler in their elbows and other skin tightening devices and have had zero luck getting the youthful-looking elbows they wanted. It got me thinking: What if I used the knowledge I have on lifts and apply it to the elbow? It worked! The great thing about an elbow lift is that it doesn't require patients to go under. We use a local anesthetic and then I carefully remove any excess skin from the elbow area.

Given how much movement we have at our elbows, this procedure needs to be done very carefully, as you don't want to remove too much skin and affect the range of motion. I put my patients in an elbow splint following the procedure to minimize movement and avoid any complications with the stitches. On average, it takes patients about eighteen months to fully heal from this surgery, and there will be scarring, which I remind my patients ahead of time so they can make an informed decision.

Keeping The Vagina Tight, Fresh & Sensitive

Moving on!

Let's not lie to ourselves. We've *all* thought about it: That our undercarriages could look a little, well…snazzier. The truth is, the labia changes as we age. Like the rest of our bodies, it can become droopier, inflamed, and, well, really less appealing overall. The good news is, there are treatments that really work when it comes to freshening up the vaginal region…

And I've done them! I underwent a full vaginal reconstruction and labiaplasty when I was in my early forties. It didn't quite go as smoothly as you'd imagine though and wasn't nearly as simple as going in for a consultation, setting up the surgery time, and eagerly waiting for the surgery day to arrive. Instead, it turned into an emergency situation, and it was so scary!

I knew I wanted things tightened up down there, so I did my research and came across Dr. Robert Moore from the Atlanta Center for Aesthetic Vaginal Surgery. He seemed like the cream of the crop, and he was! I scheduled a consultation with him for a vaginal rejuvenation. The major issues I faced were incontinence and the fact that I was so loose down there that I couldn't feel anything during sex. It was bad. And not great for my marriage.

But when Dr. Moore examined me, he was literally like, *"Oh my God!"* Turned out, I had serious internal damage and, as he described it in layman's terms, it looked like my uterus was about to drop out of me. I needed to be operated on immediately. I was terrified, to say the least, as this wasn't something I expected. I didn't even get to go home first; he insisted we do the surgery in Atlanta the very next day.

And my friends, this was no quick little surgery. The entire operation took around six hours. I ended up needing a major internal reconstruction, strictly for medical reasons. Aesthetically, Dr. Moore altered my labia, because the skin of one fold hung lower than the other. Dr. Moore was *amazing* all around—he's one of the best surgeons in the world for vaginal reconstruction. Even back in 2010, when these surgeries were fairly new, he did an amazing job.

Although the surgery went well and the results were spectacular, the recovery was the most painful of any surgery I've had. I had a catheter for two weeks after the surgery and was prescribed Percocet with Tylenol for the pain, which had the side effect of making me terribly constipated. Words cannot fully describe the pain. Since I had a catheter, I couldn't go to the bathroom, so I had to take MiraLAX. Then I would have *explosions*. I ended up needing to wear a freakin' diaper! Not to mention during that two week period, I had to go to the emergency room *three times*. My husband was in Las Vegas for much of this, so I was handling it all solo for the most part. Eventually, the doctor changed my pain medication, and that helped a lot. Once the catheter was out, I was on the mend, but everything down there hurt for a good month.

Again, I got this done all the way back in 2010. Fortunately, things are *still* looking and feeling great down there. Despite the pain in those first weeks after the surgery, I have no regrets and wouldn't trade it for anything—not just for health reasons, but also for aesthetic appearance too. I'm as tight as could be and I won't have to repeat the procedure. (It's one of those rare procedures that will actually pass the test of time. Truly lasting effects!) Now I just get some filler in the labia from time to time, and things look nice and plump.

Some women I've talked to about my experiences still believe some of the crazy myths about vaginal reconstruction, and that holds them back from doing it. I've had multiple women tell me, "I'm scared my clitoris will accidentally get chopped off during the process!" I can guarantee you, it will not. Like anything else, once you find the right doctor, you'll be in excellent hands with nothing to fear. (Keep in mind that the right doctor will have a thorough discussion with you about your medical history, concerns, and expectations to help determine if this surgery is the right choice for you.)

Tightening It Up Downtown

Okay, so let's get a little more technical. What exactly is vaginal reconstruction surgery? Vaginoplasty is a medical procedure that reshapes and tightens the vaginal canal, restoring and enhancing the structure and function of the vaginal region. This surgery can serve a medical purpose *and* a personal purpose (as it did for me) and it can also have physical and emotional benefits.

Most women feel the need for this surgery after giving birth because of the changes that result down there. For example, the vaginal tissue can become stretched and weakened, leaving behind a loss of muscle tone. Lots of women long for the vaginal tightness in the time before they had kids. Aging also contributes to loosening muscles down there. As we get older, our hormone fluctuations lead to changes in the vaginal tissues, impacting elasticity and lubrication. There are also other cases of congenital conditions that can affect the vaginal canal, or certain traumas that can cause structural issues.

During the vaginoplasty surgery, patients are put under anesthesia. The doctor will tighten the vaginal area by removing any extra tissue, repairing any visual damage, and then repositioning things as needed. You'll leave with a bit of a recovery journey ahead of you, but your lady bits will be tight and toned—plus, they'll function a whole lot better. Some women report an improved sex life after recovery thanks to the tightness and the renewed sensation down there. It's a huge confidence boost too. (You can certainly trust me on that one!)

Now on to the recovery (ugh!). Again, this is, in my opinion, the *only* downside to this surgery. But once you're recovered, it's really all worth it. My surgery was so intense and complicated that a catheter was needed, but it isn't always required. The length of recovery time will vary depending on the person, but most women can be up and feeling normal within a few weeks. However, during that time, you're encouraged to take it easy—and no sex! Also, no strenuous exercise during that recovery period.

My vaginal reconstruction surgery was expensive because it was very intense, but it can be as little as $1,400 to $4,500, depending on the complexity of the surgery.

I had my labiaplasty done at the same time as my vaginal reconstruction, but some women may only want or need one or the other. A labiaplasty will adjust the size and shape of the inner and outer vaginal lips. It's mostly aesthetic, but sometimes is done to relieve any discomfort a woman might experience down there. This surgery tends to cost between $4,000 and $6,000.

If you want to tighten things up but aren't ready for the surgical route, there are lasers that can help too, like the MonaLisa Touch, FemTouch, and FemiLift. Radiofrequency treatments can also be used, like the Thermi Va treatment.

Keeping *Her* Fresh with a Vajacial

Since my downtown area has been glowing for more than a decade, I'd like to keep her that way… nice, fresh and clean! One of the things I want to try soon—and that people say great things about— is a vaginal facial (or a "vajacial"). This is like a regular facial; except it's focused on the skin around the vulva to promote skin health.

If you're getting it done professionally, a vaginal facial starts with a gentle exfoliation to remove dead skin cells, promoting a smoother, more radiant appearance. This can involve mild exfoliants or physical exfoliation with scrubs. Then comes the moisturizing stage which helps fight any dryness of the skin. Brightening products can often be used, such as those with vitamin C or chamomile, to help give the skin a healthy and even tone. For women dealing with ingrown hairs, the facial will often include a treatment for these. (I laser my pubic hair so I don't have this issue.) If you're worried about getting irritated skin, don't be! These facials don't use any harsh ingredients, like chemicals or fragrances, given how sensitive the vulva area can be. If you're going to a professional to do it, expect the cost to be anywhere from about $75 to about $250.

If you feel a little too shy to visit a professional for this, you can give yourself a vaginal facial at home. Just follow the same basic steps as above, making sure to avoid those harsh chemicals! You don't want to cause any unnecessary problems or irritations. Because OUCH!

Whether it's removing some excess fat, enhancing your ladies, or freshening and tightening things up, remember to do what's right for you and what makes you look and feel like the best possible version of yourself! (And just because it's not the first thing staring at you in the mirror every morning, don't neglect the downstairs—it's important, too!)

PART TWO

FEELING YOUNG FROM THE INSIDE OUT

CHAPTER SEVEN

BEYOND CONVENTIONAL MEDICINE

If we're going to talk about aging, we *need* to talk about it from the inside out.

I am *all about* biohacking. What's biohacking, you might ask? It's basically the science of living a long life. It's "DIY biology," so ways of hacking your own biology to improve health and well-being. I've practiced all kinds of biohacking to feel physically, mentally, and emotionally my best. It's all done in the name of self-care, and it starts with getting the right nutrients into your body.

Let's rewind. I had a terrifying health scare when I started writing this book. I've lived a very healthy lifestyle for years, taking lots of the right vitamins and supplements so that I rarely get sick.

But then, out of nowhere, I was hit with the worst illness of my life. I couldn't figure out what was happening to me. I'd never considered this before, but I thought I was going to die.

I'd gone out to lunch with my husband one afternoon when, out of nowhere, I started to feel like crap. We left the restaurant right away, and he drove us home. By the time I got to the house and took my temperature, it was 103.9 degrees. I went to bed and slept on and off, all while sweating and feeling completely delirious. My temperature would go down to 100, then back up to 103.9, and this all went on for five days. I should have gone to the hospital right away but for some reason I was scared. It's like that fear of death became more real every time I thought of entering the hospital.

I had body aches, diarrhea, and excruciating muscle pain…even my skin hurt! Just as my fever seemed to subside, I started to have difficulty breathing, which knocked me out even more. I was completely depleted. A nurse came to my house to check on me and was shocked at how bad my levels were. I literally had people praying for me to get better, because there was no clue as to what was happening. After about a week of suffering, I started spitting up blood. I wasn't getting better at all, so I finally decided to go to the hospital. But the doctors there couldn't figure out what was wrong with me either. They took about fifteen vials of blood and sent it to an outside lab to finally get the answer: I had dengue.

I'd never even heard of dengue before. I later learned it's a viral infection that's spread through mosquito bites. And I was right…it's often deadly! Dengue is so rare that I was only the ninth case in Miami-Dade County for the year (I was diagnosed in October of 2023). That's only nine out of 2.4 million people! And there were only 1,800 documented cases in total in the entire United States. My odds of getting this were *so* low. It was crazy.

There is no treatment for dengue either. The doctors gave me a pain killer at the hospital (that I didn't use), so I had to just ride it out. Even though there is no treatment, my genius naturopathic doctor, Dr. Nadia Musavvir (www.drmusavvir.com/dr-nadia), stepped in to help me. I'm honestly blessed to have this woman in my life. She studied the blood test results from my hospital visit and used them to create a nutrient cocktail for me. For example, since my liver levels were *so bad,* Dr. Nadia based the nutrient cocktail on the nutrients I was deficient in. I immediately started injecting the nutrient cocktail into my leg every other day. And I finally started to recover. Because of Dr. Nadia and this cocktail (which I've continued to take), this is the best I've ever felt in my life. Dr. Nadia saved me, for sure!

If I hadn't committed to taking care of my body this way, I can't imagine how much longer my symptoms would have lasted. From the time I experienced my first symptom, I'd say it was about two months until I felt completely normal. I was upset, too, because I'd lost all of the muscle tone I'd worked so hard to get. I had to start all over again at the gym. But, all in all, this could have been so much worse if I hadn't gotten ahead of things.

Over our time working together, Dr. Nadia has really gotten to know me and what my body needs. She's run a range of tests, including comprehensive blood testing, micronutrient testing (this is important because the supplements you need can constantly be changing), dried urine test for comprehensive hormones, comprehensive GI stool analysis, a methylation profile, and a biological age testing kit. It's given her a great overall picture of how my body functions and what it needs.

Now Dr. Nadia and I test my blood every three months, and alter the nutrient injection based on those results. If internal wellness was a huge part of my beauty routine before, it's even more important now. So you can get a quick glance, here are the supplements I take regularly right now:

- **Every other day:** One vitamin injection that contains a mixture of the Myer's cocktail (vitamin B, vitamin C, magnesium, and calcium), Methionine Inositol Choline (MIC) to break down fat, and gluten thyrogen.
- **Every other day:** One NAD injection to boost energy, mood, and brain function.
- **Two months on, two months off, daily:** One injection of peptides CJC-1295 and GHK-Cu to help reverse aging. (The peptides are *crucial* for anti-aging!!! I'm adding extra exclamation points because that's how strongly I feel about this idea. Remember how I've said my facelift has required upkeep? The peptides are one of the primary things I use to maintain the results.)
- **Two months off, two months on:** One injection of the peptides Epitalon and Thymosin alpha 1—also to help reverse aging.

To help me keep track of everything I take, I use an app called Fullscript, which I highly recommend to anyone whose practitioner is familiar with it. Here are the other supplements I take orally every day:

- PurePaleo protein chocolate
- OmegAvail TG1000
- Biocidin Broad Spectrum
- Ultra Binder Sensitive
- ADK
- Liver-G.I. Detox
- LypoZyme
- Mag SRT
- Nanoformulated DHEA+
- MethylCare

If you're considering starting a regimen of supplements like mine, please consult with a naturopathic doctor to understand your baselines and what supplements are best for you. It's easy to just go into a drugstore and grab some supplements off a shelf to start taking. But why take stuff that isn't tailored to you? Find a naturopath!

Also, you might find that ordering vitamin injections through a naturopath can be quite pricy, so if that's the case, ask the naturopath where you can purchase the supplements on your own for less money. This can be done on a budget!

Dr. Joel Wallach founded Youngevity, a wellness company whose mission is to help people live long and feel great (he's even written books about wanting to help people live to one hundred years old—I recommend checking out him and his books). Youngevity sells all sorts of wellness-related products (essential oils, skincare) but I specifically love one of their products called 90 Essentials Nutrients. According to Dr. Wallach, there are ninety minerals that our bodies need for optimal health, and most of us don't even come close to getting enough. I drink eight ounces of this drink every day for a full serving to get all of my minerals in (warning, it doesn't have the greatest taste, so I recommend cutting it with another beverage).

I also drink one or two collagen drinks per day. I like the 1.69 ounce Isagenix Collagen Elixir drinks the best. They have five grams of collagen peptides, biotin, vitamin C, zinc, and a superfood blend of phytonutrient-rich goji and acerola berries, aloe vera, and chamomile. It's great for both the skin and the hair!

I'm a vegetarian, so finding ways to get my protein in is important for me, especially considering I enjoy weight training and being toned. A woman my weight should be getting about 43 grams of protein, but since I try to gain and maintain muscle, I aim higher.

Every morning, before my workout, I eat two Ma's Protein Snacks blueberry protein donuts, which collectively have 30 grams of protein (and are very low in sugar—another huge bonus!). They have clean ingredients too: eggs, Greek yogurt, applesauce, protein powder, egg white, coconut flour, blueberries, erythritol, cream, cheeses, sugar free maple syrup, and baking powder. And they're freakin' delicious! I then drink a protein shake throughout my workout—typically the REDCON1 MRE Protein Shake in milk chocolate, which has 40 grams of protein. This means I've hit 70 grams of protein for the day, before I've ever left the gym (I space it out throughout the workout though, so I'm not getting all 70 grams at once). I used to get only about 50 grams a day of protein and now I'm up to between 100 and 125 grams. It's made the biggest difference in my body!

Another thing I take is three grams a day of creatine and I mix it with water. Its benefits include increases muscle strength and endurance, boosts muscle hydration, improves lean muscle mass, and speeds up muscle recovery time. All of this combined, I've literally never felt better.

I feel great and I've also noticed a real change in how my body looks, especially since increasing the amount of protein I take. Everything is *tighter* everywhere on my body and I'm so much stronger than I've ever been. It's honestly been incredible to witness. In my opinion, it's never too early to meet your own Dr. Nadia and get clear on what you can and should be taking. This way you're able to be as proactive about your internal wellness as possible.

Why Holistic Medicine?

Holistic medicine is often thought of as an alternative approach to conventional medicine. A lot of people have trouble getting behind it, and I think it's because we as a society are so accustomed to conventional medicine that it's hard to consider anything else. For me, I've always hated that feeling of being just another name on a prescription pad. Being rushed in and out of doctor's appointments, with no personal connections, and often leaving more confused than anything else. On the total opposite end, I love my experience with Dr. Nadia—it's incredibly personalized.

Holistic medicine takes a far more comprehensive approach to a person's overall well-being and digs deep into what's going on inside of the person. I don't go into Dr. Nadia's office for her to say, "Oh this new vitamin is all the rage! Take it!" Instead, she works with me to make sure every single thing we put into my body is actually right for me.

Now, I'm not here to tell you to ditch your primary care physician! I don't have a medical degree, so you need to do your own research and see what's right for you. But, by nature of this entire book, I want to lay it all out there…here are some things I personally love about working with a naturopathic doctor:

- **I'm important!** I used to feel like just another name in a chart—totally irrelevant. Holistic approaches really treat me as a human being. I'm never rushed in and out the door. I get personalized care on everything from my nutrition to my stress levels.

- **I'm unique!** I don't believe symptoms should be treated with a one-size-fits-all approach. It makes no sense to me, especially because I'm a unique individual. Dr. Nadia never puts my symptoms into a box—she digs to the root cause of any health issues, so we know whatever treatment we use is right for *me*.

- **I'm in control!** This way of looking at my health has put me behind the wheel. Dr. Nadia gives me the knowledge (and the tools and strategies) to manage my own health. I'm never, ever left popping a pill while asking, *"Why am I doing this?!"*

- **I love natural alternatives!** Let's face it, Mother Nature didn't spend millions of years perfecting herbs, plants, and natural remedies for us to ignore them in favor of a little white pill. There is a ton of healing power to be found in nature and I love those alternatives.

Dr. Nadia and her husband, Shan Siddiqi (a conventional doctor), run their practice together and they're able to blend their traditional and integrative medical expertise. Dr. Nadia sees patients virtually and their in-person location helps clients focus on improving their general health as well as healthy aging.

Here is some expert insight into holistic medicine from the expert herself, Dr. Nadia.

HOLISTIC MEDICINE
Words from the Wise:
Nadia Musavvir,
Licensed Naturopathic Doctor

I always encourage people to educate themselves as early as possible about health and wellness, and to always be in the know about their bodies, diets, and overall well-being. It's so critical to be proactive.

The key difference in my approach, compared to conventional medicine, is that I work with my patients to make sure we're not just looking at an immediate treatment for a current problem or symptom, but that we're looking at the whole picture and their ongoing health and wellness journey.

I like to focus on comprehensive blood work with my patients to make sure the plan we come up with for them is tailored properly. This blood work goes well beyond what's usually done in a yearly physical panel, which often focuses on disease detection rather than overall health optimization. Conventional blood work definitely has limitations when it comes to identifying underlying health issues. For example, I've had patients come to me who were experiencing symptoms, like fatigue or skin issues, but conventional tests failed to pinpoint their root cause. By conducting a more thorough analysis, including specific markers like fasting insulin, we could uncover hidden health issues that standard panels missed.

Let's say a patient comes to me because they're experiencing unexplained hair loss—I make it my mission to get to the root cause, rather than simply prescribing them a topical treatment or surgical procedure to fix it. I want to know why this hair loss is happening. Sometimes it's lack of iron, for example, and the patient never even considered that. Chronic diseases and other internal health issues are often exhibited through hair and skin problems too, so we take a deep look at all of that. Then, once we've determined the cause, we can talk about other solutions. (Something I love for hair loss and healthy skin is PRF, Platelet Rich Fibrin, a gel for promoting hair growth and healthy aging of the skin. It's a treatment derived from the patient's own blood and I've seen a lot of people have success with it.)

I start with my new patients by reviewing their medical history and any symptoms they might be experiencing, if any. I'll then run that extensive blood work panel, which includes markers for inflammation, thyroid health, and metabolic markers. Together these provide a detailed understanding of a patient's internal health. With that in hand, we determine the nutrients they need.

Most of my patients choose to do injectable nutrients, as they can provide a faster and more effective route to address any nutrient deficiencies. Injection allows the nutrients to bypass typical ways of digestion, which maximizes the absorption. That said, injections aren't always the right option for people (some people are scared to do them, to be honest). In that case, oral supplements can absolutely be taken. It's really important to make this something that's easy and best for the patient.

You might be someone who takes a multivitamin to cover your bases, or some kind of one-size-fits-all supplement for your health needs, and there's nothing wrong with that. These types of supplements can provide a baseline, though they often fall short of meeting a person's individual requirements. Remember, there's a difference between a general formula and a clinical dose, and that personalized care tailors interventions to a person's specific needs.

Sometimes we'll have patients come to us who are prescribed a certain drug, but are hoping to go off of it and use something natural instead. In these cases, we can determine the right health interventions for an individual by gathering information on their genetics, lifestyle, and even blood type. While some people might genuinely need that prescription medication, sometimes things like lifestyle changes—including dietary modifications and exercise—might allow for reduced dosages over time. And sometimes there are natural alternatives we can offer them as well. Overprescription is so common with traditional medication because, a lot of times, doctors overlook the big picture of the patient. We make sure to take everything into account.

When I give my patients my recommendations, I trust they'll use the right supplements and make any recommended lifestyle changes if they want to see real and lasting results. I completely understand that not everyone may be ready for a total overhaul, but I believe there's a need for at least some level of commitment to see positive outcomes. Luckily, nearly all of my patients are committed, and they're living healthier lives because of it.

For the most part, clients tend to work with me for a minimum of three months, and many then choose to continue beyond that. With my long-term patients, we'll do annual blood work panels which allows for us to make any necessary adjustments to the nutrients they take. (We do Sandy's more often because of her experience with dengue, but eventually we'll stretch hers out as well).

For people who are interested in a holistic approach to health, and want to find someone in their area, I recommend seeking naturopathic doctors who have completed accredited four-year programs, and making sure they have the necessary qualifications for comprehensive care.

Holistic medicine is not often covered by insurance, but I view this as the ultimate investment in your health. (Yes, I'm biased, but I mean this!) Think of the long-term benefits and potential cost savings compared to dealing with medical issues that can come up in the future if you're not proactive. Yes, there are a lot of misconceptions about holistic medicine, but by adopting a holistic approach, people can really address the root cause of their health issues and experience tons of positive changes. And this goes beyond just treating symptoms.

Another thing to mention is this: There are so many treatments out there that people simply don't know about. Let's consider one in particular that's being used for anti-aging and treating certain diseases too. It uses the body's own stem cells to achieve results. The treatment involves removing the stem cells from the person's own body and then duplicates them. They're then injected back into the person through an IV, and those cells attack any harmful cells, while leaving the healthy cells unharmed. It's an excellent approach in that it uses the body's own natural defenses to fight both age and disease. The best part is that it's showing very promising results.

The Ohhh-Mazing O-Shot & Exosome Therapy

Another thing I do for internal wellness—and for the wellness of my freakin' sex life—is **the O-Shot**. I recently found out about the O-Shot and I'm *hooked.* It's marketed as a way to enhance female pleasure, and boy oh boy does it achieve that. The process is fairly simple and is usually done by a nurse or nurse practitioner: A small amount of blood is drawn from your arm. A machine then spins the blood sample to isolate the platelet-rich plasma (PRP). (The PRP has certain growth factors that play a role in tissue repair and regeneration.) After the PRP has been isolated, a numbing cream is applied to the vagina. Once everything is numb down there, a needle then injects the PRP into the clitoris and upper vagina. This has the effect of re-generating tissue, increasing blood flow, and im-proving sexual function.

Speaking from experience, I've experienced in-creased sensation, increased natural lubrication, and waaaaay better orgasms! Overall sexual func-tion is at a peak. I started getting the O-Shot in my fifties. It lasts about a year or two, depending on the person. While you might think the injection would hurt, the numbing cream reduced any potential pain so all you'll really feel during the procedure is a bit more pressure than anything else. When it comes to pricing, you can expect to pay somewhere between $1,200 and $2,500 for the shot.

Exosome therapy is something I'm about to try too. It's excellent for anti-aging since it's shown to have an ability to promote collagen and elastin production, promote tissue rejuvenation, and enhance skin health. It's also now being used to treat hair loss and it has a ton of other health benefits: injury treatment, treating neurodegenerative diseases like Alzheimer's, Parkinson's, and stroke-related damage, help for patients with autoimmune diseases, like rheumatoid arthritis, lupus, and multiple sclerosis, repairing damaged heart tissue and improving cardiac function, reducing inflammation, and a lot more.

Exosomes are released by cells in the body, and they contain important components, including proteins and DNA (these play roles in cell growth and communication). Exosomes basically carry "instructions" and travel between cells to influence how they behave—they can tell cells to do things like grow, repair themselves, and fight off infections. So, exosomes are very important in maintaining overall cellular health.

Though the process can vary depending on where someone receives exosome therapy, for me, I prefer to have my doctor draw my blood and send it to a lab where exosomes can be extracted and purified. A lot of times the purified exosomes will be injected into a patient using an IV treatment, but you might remember from Chapter 1 that I absolutely *HATE* IVs after my experience with them left me incredibly swollen and puffy. (The saline in them is a huge NO for me!) So, instead my doctor is going to inject the exosomes directly into my skin. I'm really excited to see the results.

If you're interested in this treatment, keep in mind that it can get expensive—usually starting at $2,000 per treatment, and it's not covered by most insurance plans. (A lot of places charge about $10,000 per treatment, so shop around—and make sure you're seeing someone who is professionally trained to do this!)

Sorry, It Must Just Be the Hormones!

As women, our ongoing hormonal changes can really mess with our health and wellness. When I was in my forties and going through menopause I honestly needed some relief. I was having symptoms—like hot flashes and mood swings that I genuinely couldn't control. But worst of all was the vaginal dryness during sex; it was bad to the point where it was unbearably painful.

I kept hearing about the success women had with Hormone Replacement Therapy (HRT) and I wanted the same relief. I made an appointment at my gynecologist's office, and she gave me the rundown: Hormone Replacement Therapy involves taking medication—both oral and topical—to replenish the estrogen that the body stops producing during menopause and perimenopause. My takeaway from the appointment was that taking HRT would cause my symptoms to subside. So I said, "Sign me up!"

Within a couple of months, I noticed the vaginal dryness going away, which was huge. Beyond the initial benefits I experienced, I learned that HRT can also improve bone health by preventing bone loss and can reduce the risk of osteoporosis in postmenopausal women. There are cognitive benefits, too, such as improved memory and mental clarity. And it can increase libido, boost your energy, and improve your mood (this one was the exact OPPOSITE for me!).

BUT! What I wasn't prepared for was that estrogen causes an increase in hyperpigmentation. So, my sunspots I fought forever were giving me more of a problem than ever. I was so mad! The estrogen also made me…like, *mean*! My personality changed—it was as if I was possessed by a demon at times. My injector, Denise Santoli, even called me out on it after I sent her some rage texts one day. I'm laughing typing that because it was just that out of control!

Ultimately, I decided to come off it, and I'll personally never do HRT again. But plenty of women have great experiences with it, so I wouldn't write it off if you're having bad symptoms.

Here are the hormones that are usually included:

- **Estrogen:** Frequently used in women experiencing menopausal symptoms like hot flashes, vaginal dryness, and mood swings.
- **Progesterone**: Often prescribed along with estrogen to protect the uterus lining and alleviate symptoms.
- **Testosterone:** Administered to address symptoms of low testosterone, which can affect both men and women.
- **Thyroid Hormones:** Used to regulate thyroid function and address conditions like hypothyroidism.

Given how much our hormones impact our body, it's important to talk to your doctor about any risks that might come with HRT before you start treatment. Some of the more severe risks include blood clots, strokes, and breast cancer. So, check with your doctor to make sure this is a viable option for you before you start.

If you do decide to try HRT, keep in mind that your doctor will want to schedule regular check-ups to make sure the treatment is effective and to make any adjustments. This is a very good thing!

You'll learn to pay attention to your body and to always listen to what it tells you—kind of like how mine was telling me *hell no!* If new symptoms pop up while you're undergoing HRT, and you didn't have these symptoms before, let your doctor know ASAP.

For me, I've seen what works best is solely taking testosterone. I also use the Glutaryl spray ($119.95) an antioxidant spray that contains high doses of glutathione (while glutathione is not a hormone, it does aid in hormonal balance). Glutathione promotes cellular health, helps eliminate toxins from the body, and helps improve immunity, detoxification, energy levels, and anti-aging. I spray it on my stomach twice a day.

The Price to Pay for Living Well

As Dr. Nadia mentioned, insurance usually doesn't cover holistic medicine. So, you might be wondering what this type of treatment will set you back. Naturopathic doctors usually do an initial consultation for between $100 and $300, which includes the first round of blood work. Follow-up visits can run around $100 to $200. If the doctor recommends any treatments for you, those costs can really be all over the map.

Again, this is really the best way to get a complete picture of what's going on in your body. You can treat symptoms but also be incredibly proactive too. I love that naturopathic doctors aren't just writing out any ol' prescription. Think of how many medications you've probably taken in your lifetime that you really didn't need! OMG, so many! I don't know about you, but something just doesn't sit right with me about that.

It doesn't sit right with my close friend, Monica Hart, either. She is another patient of Dr. Nadia's who started working with her because she wanted to come off any unnecessary medications she was on. She's had a real awakening in recent years and now swears by holistic medicine.

Here are some of her insights on the topic.

HOLISTIC MEDICINE
Words from the Wise: Monica Hart

During the COVID-19 pandemic I had an epiphany of sorts. I didn't trust the narratives being told to us, and it got me thinking more about healthcare as a whole, and what we're blindly asked to accept about our own personal health and wellness. Suddenly, nothing made sense to me. This is really when I became very mindful of what things I was putting into my body, and that included medications as well as foods and nutrients.

I began to research a lot about Western medicine, and found it's completely hijacked. There is just so much misinformation out there. This realization led me to embrace holistic medicine, and I started to work with Dr. Nadia, who approached everything we talked about with an open mind and a commitment to uncovering the truth too.

One medication that stuck out to me in my research is statin, which is used to lower cholesterol. I found that many years ago, the medical community altered the standard cholesterol values to promote the widespread use of this drug. This means many, many patients are being prescribed this who don't actually need it. It's scary! Not only that, but contrary to popular belief, these medications can contribute to a ton of health issues, like neurological conditions and even cancer. By looking at their health holistically instead, many patients can come off this medication, avoid those risks, and feel just as good and healthy. I always encourage people to find natural remedies over pharmaceutical interventions.

(If you ever have time, look into the Rockefeller family's influence on all of this. They had vested interests in the medical industry that have shaped mainstream narratives and perpetuated a cycle of illness and dependency.)

After working with Dr. Nadia, I started making some significant changes personally. I learned a few years ago that I have celiac disease which means I cannot consume gluten. Again, I did a ton of research into this, and learned none of us—celiac or not—need gluten in our diets. I'm a proponent of a gluten-free lifestyle for everyone. This is just one way I've started to reclaim my health. I am also now mindful of the toxins that are built up in all of our bodies. I do regular colon cleanses and liver cleanses on occasion as well.

Being healthy from the inside out means not relying on conventional medicine to merely manage symptoms. You want to be proactive. You'd be surprised to know how many seemingly unrelated ailments are actually connected. (For example, I've learned there is a connection between dental health and chronic conditions. If a person has metal in their mouth, whether through a root canal, fillings, or anything else, it can lead to chronic illness.)

I cannot stress enough the importance of critical thinking and questioning the status quo. Do your own research and have conversations with a naturopathic doctor and you'll be able to take control of your own health and well-being. Ask questions, seek out alternative perspectives, and trust your own intuition. It definitely requires both courage and curiosity, but it'll put you in the driver seat of your own health.

Now that I view my health holistically, I'll never look back. It makes me feel good to know I'm doing everything I can to make sure the inside of my body is feeling just as young as the outside looks! But, as you know, internal wellness goes well beyond what you're putting into your body. It's also about your emotional well-being too. In the next chapter, we'll talk all about what I do to stay mentally well (it's been a challenge at times, don't get me wrong). I'm about to unveil a whole aspect of my life that has challenged my mental wellness countless times over the years.

CHAPTER EIGHT

MIND VERSUS AGE

We all have triggers that make us feel scared or anxious, am I right? I bet that just by reading that sentence, you were able to come up with a whole laundry list of your own triggers. Family issues, money, work, lack of sleep, that laundry piling up (speaking of!) …I can go on and on. But what happens when that anxiety starts to impact our daily lives? It weighs on us…and Hell! Makes us feel tired and freakin' OLD.

Stress and anxiety also cause wrinkles!! What's the good of getting poked and prodded with wrinkle relaxers if we're just going to cause more wrinkles by worrying. What we think matters as much as how we look. And I'm not just talking about, "Oh, my mindset is that age is just a number!" Well, yes, it is. And that's a great reminder to yourself. But there's more to this whole concept of *thinking younger.*

To rewire my brain, I had to take a slightly less conventional route at first.

What I Gained from Ibogaine

I'm not a particularly anxious person overall. I don't typically overthink situations or imagine worst-case scenarios, though I know plenty of women who do. But I have some anxiety triggers that impact my own daily life—such as…elevators.

Elevators scare the crap out of me! I hate how small the space inside that little box is, and even the thought of sharing it with other people freaks me out. Not to mention the idea that an elevator can get stuck any second, and then I'm trapped in there. *AHHH!* It freaks me out to even write it on the page!

I refuse to take the elevator unless I'm sure—*like 100 percent sure!* —that there is an elevator maintenance worker present in the building. Imagine how much this impacts my life here in Miami, where there are *so many* high-rises! For example, when I visit Johanna Hedman for my microblading appointments, I use the stairs every time, even though her office is on the sixteenth floor. There is no way I'm getting on that elevator. One time I even climbed fifty-seven flights of stairs to avoid an elevator. Fifty-seven! Even though I work out a lot, that is A LOT of steps!

I have tried therapy, medication, and hypnosis, all to no avail. I've also tried some mind-opening drugs like Ayahuasca as well. (I haven't tried others like DMT, Bufo, or psilocybin, but I know people have found help in those.) Then I heard about ibogaine. (At first, I thought it sounded more like the name of a sci-fi movie than an anxiety cure, but what did I know?) Ibogaine is a psychedelic drug derived from the roots of the African iboga plant. It's used in some places outside of the United States as a treatment for drug addiction and also for people with PTSD. But when it's not used to treat addiction, ibogaine, in smaller doses, can also be used to help people change behavioral patterns and put life into perspective. Essentially, it's been super-effective in rewiring the brain, and that was exactly what I needed! I was ready for a nonconventional path.

Ibogaine can only be administered in a specialized clinic under medical supervision. You should also be aware that this experience might take you into the deep, dark parts of your mind. There are medical risks—such as a slowed heart rate, a decrease in blood pressure, seizures, trouble breathing—which is why supervision is a must. The costs vary, but the one-time Ibogaine treatment for anxiety at a supervised clinic will usually run between $4,000 and $15,000.

I heard once from a trusted source about a clinic in Mexico that administers ibogaine in a safe, controlled setting. So, I figured, what the heck! I'll try it. While at the clinic, a facilitator monitors the patient while you're undergoing the experience, so I wasn't scared to do it.

IBOGAINE WARNING: Before we go any further, I am by no means advocating this for *your* mental health. I'm only telling you about *my* own experience. If you ever decide to try ibogaine for yourself, then please, please, *please* do your research and find the right clinic. There <u>must</u> be a facilitator in there with you. When my husband tried ibogaine, his heart rate dropped significantly during the treatment. Thankfully, he went to the same clinic I did, and his facilitator was able to return his heart rate to a safe range. So, if you're going to do it (and do it safely), be prepared! Your journey could be slightly terrifying, but it will definitely be enlightening. An excellent facility our close friends George and Diane run in Cabo San Lucas, Mexico is The POI Institute. You can learn more about their facility, who they help, and what they offer at www.poiibogaine.com or by calling 1-833-764-2226.

Now for my experience. I'll be real: It was *crazy!* But crazy in a good way. I knew that I would have visions while in a psychedelic state. I just didn't realize that my entire life would flash before my eyes—it was VERY vivid, too! And it wasn't all the good stuff; I saw some awful things from my childhood.

Here's how it worked: When I got to the clinic, the facilitator handed me a capsule with the drug and an eye mask. They told me to wear the eye mask, but that I could remove it at any time to decrease the visions (which was comforting). I took the medication and laid down on a bed in the facility to wait for the effects. Ibogaine opens access to ten times more of your brain than is typically available, so I saw flashes of my life that I had never remembered previously. It felt like I was watching a movie of my life that had somehow tapped into the depths of my subconscious.

A lot of it had to do with my childhood. My sister and I are both adopted—I was adopted as a baby from Baltimore and my sister was adopted from Korea. We both went to live with our adoptive parents in the suburbs of Baltimore, Maryland. We were an upper-middle class family and we seemed to have had a very normal childhood. But clearly there were things that my brain had blocked out. My biological mother popped up in some of these memories as the Wicked Witch. Her face was haunting. I knew growing up that she wasn't the best person—my adoptive parents were honest with me about her—but now it was all even clearer.

Then there was a flashback of the worst moment in my childhood—one I already knew happened, but now here it was in crystal-clear detail. I rode horses as a kid. One day my dad was late to pick me up from my riding lessons. I was only seven years old at the time. This is not the place or time for details, but the male riding instructor backed me into a corner in the stable and molested me. The shame I felt ate me alive. I didn't relish reliving it on ibogaine.

The drug treatment lasted about four hours, and when it wore off, a lot of things made sense. More importantly, my fear of elevators—of being in a tight space and feeling trapped with no way out— also made sense.

Ibogaine didn't cure my anxiety, but it did help me to become more aware of my behaviors, and thought patterns, and the reasons behind them. Overall, I'm grateful for the experience. My only regret is not using what I learned and immediately finding a therapist or a great life coach. I should have done the work right then and there.

Fortunately, I did a few years later. After some trouble in my marriage (more on that in the next chapter), I decided to do the work on myself with the help of a life coach. I'm still scared of elevators, and I might always be, but I've learned to nurture my inner child in other ways.

It's Time for a Life Coach!

I met renowned life coach Peter Ishkhans (www.echoingjoy.com) through a friend and I immediately liked his unique method to life coaching. Traditionally, a life coach uses goal-oriented methods to help their clients achieve their stated aspirations, such as a change in career life. But Peter's approach is different; he encourages his clients to connect with their inner selves, becoming more mindful about how they respond to external circumstances as well as the people in their lives. So, instead of letting the external world dictate how we live and feel, we base our decision making on our intuition instead.

It's genius!

Peter has an interesting backstory. He was married and living in Los Angeles working as a hair stylist. He had his own salon with tons of A-list celebrity clients; he cohosted E!'s *Fashion Police;* he even had his own TV show on The Style Network called *Peter Perfect.* Then, his marriage sadly fell apart and he up and moved to India. Peter lived in India for many years, where he spent a lot of time studying Eastern thinking. He found it to be quite different from how we think here in the West.

What Peter learned from his time in India is that our thoughts shape our reality. So, negative thoughts can prevent our personal growth and happiness. Positive self-talk is the core of what Peter teaches. His philosophy is based on self-kindness as a whole and working with him has absolutely increased how kind I am to myself. Since I've met Peter, I practice positive self-talk every day. I've noticed how it's really reshaped my life.

In our early sessions, Peter asked me to tap into my childhood self to see if any of my adult behaviors were rooted there (of course, they were). After we had that on the table, Peter continued to work with me so that I could stop living in fear of the things I couldn't control, and keep my mind focused on being kind to myself instead.

At this point, I'll have Peter explain his methods, though, since he is the expert!

MENTAL HEALTH
Words from the Wise:
Peter Ishkhans, Life Coach

Every person has experienced some sort of childhood trauma, whether they realize it or not. Now, trauma doesn't always have to mean something like abuse or abandonment. Sometimes it's something as simple as how they were disciplined that has created a certain thought pattern that a person then uses as an adult, out of habit. When I start working with a new client, I try to get them to tap into what that trauma might be.

My goal is to get my clients to change whatever thought patterns they have that are holding them back from a very happy life. Our thoughts shape our reality. Negative thoughts hinder personal growth and happiness. By practicing positive self-talk every day—and being really kind to themselves in general—people can reshape their lives and have the best experience possible.

Think about it—not many people are used to speaking to themselves in a kind manner. Often people are very hard on themselves, and they also allow the outside world to impact their self-perception. But what if they didn't? What if they took the mentality of "What that person thinks of me is their business!" instead of dwelling on it? They'd be almost immediately happier.

Now, I'm realistic that this transformation in how a person thinks won't happen overnight. Consider that you've been used to thinking a certain way for decades, it's going to be very hard to change that. But the trick is repetition—in waking up every day and practicing that positive self-talk, and then doing it again the next day, and the following day.

As my clients start to practice positive self-talk every day, I also put them on a "no complaining diet." This is exactly what you'd imagine—they can't complain. If a complaint comes into their mind, they better get rid of the thought, and under no circumstance should they speak it aloud. If they find there is something to complain about, I encourage them to find the positive in that situation. It might be hard to see at first, but it's there. This gets them switching their thoughts from negative ones to positive ones. Again, this takes repetition to get the hang of it, but the exercise is worthwhile.

A significant portion of life's challenges can be eliminated if you stop complaining. Complaining only perpetuates negativity and hinders personal growth. By adopting a "no complaining" mindset, my clients can break free from the cycle of discontent and create a more positive, harmonious life.

Life coaching should not be about imposing external narratives and pushing a "one-size-fits-all" model for people to live by. Instead, it should be about the individual person, their life story, and how they view and react to the world.

Little changes like this can bring about results very quickly. Suddenly, they will find their lives feel a lot more positive and harmonious. Things that used to make them angry are no longer even on their radar. Negative thoughts that were prone to show up before do so less and less now. They're finding happiness and peace! They're living their lives for themselves, by their means, without everything in the outside world impacting them.

Many times, people forget their own true nature. My job is to get my clients to reconnect with their inner selves—their divinity. Life's true power isn't just in achieving their goals, but recognizing and owning who they are from within. I aim to get clients to shift that focus from external circumstances to internal understanding. This empowers them a great deal.

To start to shift your mindset, consider finding a life coach who's aligned with this teaching method where we promote self-awareness. Things you can do on your own to practice this mind shift include meditation and journaling. I stress the need for consistent effort and practice since changing your thought patterns will only come from repetition. What you're really doing is reshaping your subconscious mind.

Life coaching has made me mentally stronger than ever and I've noticed my anxiety decrease because of it. I'm less stressed, and I don't let things bug me like I once did. I know *I* am the one in control of how I react to things. And the nonexistent worry lines on my face are equally thankful for it!

Make New Friends, Ditch the Old

Well, okay, I don't really mean *ditch* your old friends, not necessarily…but I'm a big proponent of cleaning house to keep yourself feeling good. Listen, toxic friends can bring us down. Often, they're the people we've been tied to for so long that we feel bad distancing from them. Like that childhood "best friend" who constantly makes digs at you? Say bye!

For example, Peter is big on how we respond to external circumstances and people. So, if we follow his way of teaching, then there is no such thing as negative people…only negative ways of responding to them. How we react is always within our own control.

That said, from my perspective, it also helps to spend less time with friends who don't bring you joy. My goal in life now is to only keep close friends who really love each other's company and bring each other only good vibes. No bad blood, no bad feelings.

During the COVID-19 pandemic I started to weed out some of the "bad seeds" in my life. Being around people who drained my energy and dampened my spirits left me feeling more exhausted than a day at the DMV. I took a hard look around at the company I kept and decided to ditch the drama. I was done with cliques, gossipers, and social hierarchies. That nonsense was so high school! So, I set some boundaries with the culprits. Then I found the ladies who lifted me up, who supported me, and who brought the good energy…and I spent more time with them.

If you feel drained by the people around you, there might be some friends you can do without. Here's a list of the kinds of friends you might want to set some boundaries with (or leave behind, if you can):

- The Convenient Friend who only reaches out when they need something.
- The Narcissist who won't stop talking about themselves.
- The Drama Queen whose always in an emergency!
- The Debbie Downer who never has anything good to say to you or anyone else.

Today, every friend I have is someone who brings freakin' *happiness* into my life. They're the people who have my back, who make me laugh until I cry, who listen, and who celebrate my successes. And I do the same for them!

Of course, there will always be people you can't eliminate from your life—like coworkers and family members. To deal with them, I've leaned heavily on what Peter has taught me—be in control of my reactions.

MENTAL HEALTH
Words from the Wise:
Peter Ishkhans, Life Coach

I want my clients to take responsibility for their own lives and the thoughts they have, rather than become a victim of their circumstances, or the people around them. If they stop caring what others do and say—by taking a "that's a reflection of them, not me" standpoint instead—they'll be so much happier and carefree for it. They can become true owners of their own spirit.

The more aware a person is of their thoughts, the better their ability to respond to the external events thrown at them in life. All of this gives people a deeper understanding of themselves and their lives and leads them to inner peace.

Let's consider the people in your life who you might consider "toxic." The only reason they're toxic is because you're giving them that power. Their power is influenced by your own thinking! The great thing is that you have a personal choice about whether to engage with them or not. If it's someone you have to have in your life, let's say a relative or a coworker, someone who you can't choose to just eliminate from your life, then change your mindset about them. They're only toxic if you think so. Redefine those relationships by changing your perspective. It's another excellent way to regain control over your emotional well-being.

A book I recommend reading is The Four Agreements by Don Miguel Ruiz. The author breaks down four foundational principles for navigating life: Be impeccable with your word, don't make assumptions, don't take anything personally, and always do your best. These principles offer a roadmap for conscious living and can significantly impact your personal and professional relationships—I've seen it firsthand.

Getting Focused

The work I've done with Peter has brought me to such a great place in terms of how I react to the world and people around me. Then, the work I've been doing with another life coach, Anna Lubavin (@annalbvn on Instagram) has helped me get really focused on specific life and business goals. As I was writing this book, for example, I realized how important an active and engaging social media account would be to show my readers what the different treatments and practices I do to look and feel young actually *look* like. I wanted to get serious about posting to my Instagram account (@SandraLenaSilverman). I knew it would be a lot of work, but I was determined.

In came Anna! She's been so vital in helping me set goals and actually achieve them. Here is her take on goal setting:

GOAL SETTING
Words from the Wise:
Anna Lubavin, Life Coach

A lot of people set goals for themselves and think once that goal is achieved, then something will change in their life. They're hoping to achieve a certain emotion when it's accomplished, when they should instead focus on how to achieve that emotion every step of the way.

The problem is, often people are disconnected from their emotions, and they don't even realize it. They think they're not achieving something simply because they need more knowledge. The approach I use with my clients is to get them to go beyond their thoughts and deeper than their feelings. I encourage them to get to a state where their inner spirit and inner drive are coming out. This helps them to figure out what goals and emotions they really want for themselves, instead of being influenced by society or having that," I'll be happy when..." mentality. People sometimes don't understand what they want until they are able to do this. They fear connecting to their emotions and feelings in this moment, so they let outside forces drive what they think their goals should be.

I do a lot of work with my clients to tap into their creative energy and eliminate their limiting beliefs and this sometimes requires exercises. From my perspective, there isn't one set of tools that applies to everyone. Going into a session with a new client, it's a mystery for me as well, because everyone is so unique, and that's the whole point. My approach is to encourage my clients to be themselves and practice a lot of self-reflection to understand what they really want—and why.

Once they've established what they're looking for, I encourage them to be mindful to act differently in the present moment (feel the emotions they're eager to feel). I tell them to not allow themselves to live out of fear. We're all the creator of our own reality. That's the main goal in life—creating what we want. It's going to bring you power to choose each moment. You should be setting goals for yourself because everything you need is inside of you.

I push my clients to work on both the present as well as the future. When they start experiencing changes in the current moment, it's amazing. I'm always very impressed by clients who are able to achieve results very fast—it's usually those with a lot of willpower, and Sandy is a great example of that.

These days, I'm the happiest I've ever been! A lot of it is thanks to the time I took to figure out my past, address it, and change my thought patterns for the future.

CHAPTER NINE:

PSYCHIC WISDOM FOR ENDURING LOVE

I don't think anything can take years off your life quite like marital troubles. I've mentioned my husband, Dave, a few times in earlier chapters, but I haven't really let you in on our marriage yet. The truth is we're separated right now… for the fourth time. (You might be thinking, "Sheesh, Sandy, I thought I knew almost everything about you at this point! I even know details about your vagina, for God's sake!" But yes, there is even more to share.)

Things Aren't Always Sweet

I knew very early on in our relationship that I was going to marry Dave, and I've worked very hard to make our marriage last. But it's been difficult.

Dave and I met in our twenties. It was August 1997, and we were out at a cigar bar in Baltimore, where we both lived then. I was dating another guy at the time, but it didn't stop Dave from telling me, "I think we would have cute kids together." (Boy, was he right!) As soon as I was single, Dave and I started dating. Both of us were doing well in our careers when we decided to start our own mortgage company together: NFM Lending. A year later, we were working together *and* living together, *and* we were engaged.

Business was booming, but the relationship… not so much.

The truth was, I brought some childhood issues into the relationship. Things started to get rocky, and during our engagement, we decided to take a break. But just like Ross and Rachel from *Friends,* each of us took the term "break" to mean something entirely different. It was a mess; I'll leave it that. We were able to move past it, got back together, and got married in August of 1999.

On the surface, people might think things have been great for us for the past 25 years. But it's actually been a roller coaster. At times things have been amazing. Then other times things have been terrible. Neither of us have been angels—we've both been at fault for different reasons, and there has been infidelity on both ends. I've made some big mistakes and so has he, and trust has been broken at certain points. Every one of our separations has been very painful.

In the bad times, we tried everything: personal development programs, counseling, life coaching. Some of it helped temporarily. Some of it didn't help at all. We simply weren't connecting the way we were supposed to.

Maybe worst of all, at one point Dave started talking to a hack who positioned herself as a certified life coach/therapist but had zero credentials. Instead of encouraging him to work on himself and our marriage and to do some introspective work, she told him to leave me for good. She said that once the connection is gone in a marriage, you can never go back. I often thought about reaching out to this woman (I won't say her name here, though I'd love to!) to tell her that she had *a lot* of nerve coaching Dave to not come home. It took everything in my power not to—I had to constantly calm myself down! And he was paying her…wait for this…$1,000 an hour, with no real credentials, to give him this awful advice.

The ups and downs caused a lot of confusion. I never knew what would happen next. I struggled with a lack of emotional security, always in fear of whether Dave would leave again or ask for a divorce. It's been tough on my mental health.

Fast forward to now. At first, I was devastated to be separated again. I cried a lot and made tons of calls to family and friends for support (I'm SO thankful to all of them!). Even though I was really upset, I decided to make a commitment to work on myself and my goals. Instead of letting the separation destroy me, I finished my first book! I stayed focused on the many good things in my life instead of the one part that was going wrong. I was still sad, but this wasn't going to leave me a shattered mess!

I also brought in another expert to guide me in feeling my best, whether that's with or without Dave. She's a gem of a human who knows *everything* ---my trusted psychic, Priscilla Keresey (www.apracticalpsychic.com).

In Your Future, I See…

I know for a fact that I wouldn't have made it through the constant uncertainties in my relationship without Priscilla. When I didn't know whether I was coming or going, she'd set me straight. Priscilla offers me clarity and guidance at every turn. (If you're someone who doesn't believe in psychic abilities, that's all fine and well. But before I lose you, let me say that if you find the right psychic—someone who is *not* a scam artist—you're going to love the experience.)

Priscilla is always there to help me understand if I'm making the right choices about my marriage. The reassurance she gives me is a total game changer! Being in the constant *unknown* of a roller coaster relationship takes its toll, but I lean on Priscilla to relieve a lot of that uneasiness now.

I found Priscilla through a friend, and I now talk to her about once a week. She's literally never been wrong with her predictions. While the cost for a good psychic can run over $200 an hour, it's worth it if it's someone like Priscilla.

BEWARE: Sometimes phonies or scammers will charge you thousands of dollars or more if they catch you in a vulnerable state of mind. I met one psychic in Los Angeles during a separation from Dave who saw me upset and then predicted Dave would ask me to dinner. There was no way I believed him. I paid and left. Then…the dinner invite actually happened! I was shocked! I knew this psychic was talented, but what I didn't know was that he was the ultimate scam artist. He kept telling me he needed to rid me of negative energy if I wanted my marriage to work. And it would cost me. The worst part is, I kept paying! It wasn't until he came to visit me in Miami and wanted $10,000 that I finally woke up!

Here is Priscilla's take on what a psychic should (and should not!) do:

PSYCHIC READINGS
Words from the Wise:
Priscilla Keresey, Psychic Medium

I started many years ago in hypnosis, helping women with food issues, and I discovered my natural ability to connect with clients on a deeper level. I became very tuned into people, so I began my work as a psychic medium. I've grown my client base since then and now have lots of clients who come to me on a regular basis, as Sandy does, for insight into their lives. Some I'll talk to monthly or even weekly, and there's a range of topics they'll be interested in, sometimes insights into their business, or their love life, or their family and friends. I also see one-time clients who come for fun or for some guidance and recommendations.

For a new client, I'll often start with a tarot card reading to get to know each other. With my long-term clients, I don't usually use tarot cards, because I've already gotten to know them well enough (though I will pull cards for them if they'd like, as Sandy usually does). Most readings are done in either a half hour, 45-minute, or hour-long session.

Psychics are able to use their own sixth sense, as well as the client's sixth sense, to determine future outcomes. My sixth sense allows me a glimpse into a person's past, present, and future. I use this to give my clients insight they can use in a practical way to make informed decisions in their life. Clients often ask me specific questions, and my readings provide another channel of information for them to use— together with their own intuition—to make those informed decisions. However, I don't make definitive predictions on very sensitive matters, like health or legal issues.

I'll provide validation for their instincts and shed light on situations. Even if the information I'm telling somebody isn't what they want to hear, they should always leave feeling empowered. I think what my clients find most often is peace of mind. Whether the answer to their questions or concerns are what they want to hear or not, at least they have some sort of clarity.

I like to remind my clients that timing in any reading will not always be exact. It's tough to say a certain thing will happen in an exact timeframe. This is because time simply doesn't work like that in another realm. I also remind my clients of an important concept: free will. Just because I may see something in a reading doesn't mean a person doesn't have the power to change that if they choose to.

I also work as a medium to connect with spirits and deliver messages from the other side. When it comes to the spirit realm, a medium can bridge the gap between the living and the dead, and offer peace and closure to people who are looking for connection to their loved one. The spirit who will show up during the reading is the spirit who has the easiest time connecting. So it's not always necessarily going to be the deceased person the client was closest to.

Not all people who first come through my door are open to the process, whether it's a psychic reading or connecting with a loved one who's passed. I definitely have clients from time to time who are skeptical, nervous, and/or resistant. Maybe they've had a negative experience with a psychic in the past which makes them not very trusting of the process. The more open a person's mindset is to the reading, and the more trusting they are, the better I can connect with them. That open mindset allows the reading to be more successful overall.

There are plenty of scammers out there who will prey on those who are vulnerable and seeking guidance. We call them "sidewalk psychics," who usually promise to do things like rid you of your "negative energy" by charging a very large fee. Be careful not to fall into these scams. If anybody ever tells you you're "cursed," or you have to pay more or buy a candle or do some sort of "healing," don't believe it!

My best advice for finding the right psychic medium for you is to go by word of mouth, like friends and family, or online reviews. Transparency, honesty, and ethical conduct are attributes I'd look for in a reputable psychic medium.

Putting Myself First

Now where was I with Dave? Ah, yes, separated…! I'm separated and focusing on *me*!

I understand the importance of compromise in a marriage, and I also understand the significance of putting work into a marriage. I did that for 25 years and I'm very proud of myself for it! But now, in this current separation – and with ongoing guidance and assurance from Priscilla that I'm following the right path – I'm putting myself first. Making myself a priority for once has made me happier than I've been in a long time. A lot of times, as women, we forget to prioritize our own mental health, especially when we're going through trouble in our relationships. It's so easy to put everyone else's needs ahead of our own. I've learned that, for me, part of feeling good overall is having the right mindset and trusted experts to guide and reassure me. I gave myself the time to focus on me and my thoughts and get my mind moving in a positive place.

I once thought I needed to stick it out with Dave no matter what, even at the expense of my own happiness. But now I've realized that my own happiness matters! I've also realized that there is nothing wrong with choosing myself. I spend a lot of time, money, and effort to look good – I want to make sure I'm prioritizing feeling good, too, in every aspect of my life!

If you're experiencing a rough patch in your own relationship, or you're heading towards a breakup or divorce, please know that you're not alone. So many couples go through it, and there's nothing to be ashamed of, or defeated by. Sometimes with the necessary work, things will work out. Sometimes, they won't. But, trust me, you can never go wrong by making yourself a priority in all of this.

(I have a lot more to share about this topic and my second book will cover it all! Stay tuned…!)

CHAPTER TEN

DRESSING THE PART

Now let's talk fashion and looking the part of a young lady! I love clothes as much as the next woman, and not just because I have an interest in fashion. It's because I know clothes have real power when it comes to aging a person, or making them feel timeless—on the outside and the inside.

Yep, you read that right: The right clothes (and jewelry, for that matter) can help us look *and* feel younger!

Don't believe me? Think back to that popular TV show from the early 2000s called *What Not to Wear.* The two hosts would overhaul someone's closet and make them get rid of anything dated, bland, and ill-fitting. (The person getting the closet makeover often didn't take this well—sometimes they'd even *cry* during the cleanout—like, *what the f*&k!)* The best part was when the hosts sent the person to shop for new pieces. After some help with hair and makeup, too, the person would always end up looking so much younger by the end of the episode.

So, like I said, clothes matter! Even if you've been doing everything right for your skin and body to look hot and young, the wrong clothes can totally ruin it all. Not only will you look older to the people around you (ick!), but you'll also feel older (double ick!).

From Rags to Riches

Reversing your age with clothes starts by simply becoming more aware. If you're someone who skims through a closet of ratty and bland clothes every morning, choosing any ol' thing to throw on, THIS IS YOUR WAKEUP CALL! Hello, it's me, Sandy, and I am sounding the alarm. Snap out of it! It's time to refresh that closet!

I work with an extremely talented personal shopper and stylist named Danielle Klein (@styledbydanielleklein on Instagram). The first session we had together, we cleaned out my closet.

Geez did it make a difference! Before Danielle, I always felt like I had an overflowing closet, yet nothing to wear. I didn't realize just how much junk I had in there—a ton of things that were just worn out and gross—until she and I went through it, piece by piece.

A lot of the clothes in my closet didn't serve me well *at all*, not only in terms of style, but also fit. I put my trust in Danielle to decide what should go and what should stay. (And, no, I didn't cry!) We donated everything in the "no" pile and came up with a plan of closet staples to buy for a youthful, timeless, and chic wardrobe.

If you're over forty, what items from your closet should you toss? According to Danielle, *very* distressed jeans and *very* skinny jeans should go. Say goodbye to ultra low-rise jeans and micro-mini bandeau dresses. For that matter, add any super short skirt to the "go" pile (they're like tequila shots: fun in your twenties, regrettable in your forties.) Sure, you want to show off those legs, but save it for home! And while Air Jordan high-tops might be all the rage with Millennials and Gen Z, can you *really* pull them off? Likely not. (But all-white hi-tops? Hell yes!)

Also, if it's frumpy, it's time to go. You know the ones—those silhouettes that do nothing for your figure except make you look like you've embraced the muumuu lifestyle. (Newsflash: shapelessness is not a good look on anyone, regardless of age.)

Okay now. Your closet's a blank slate. What should you be shopping for? Danielle helped me mix and match pieces, ranging from expensive to affordable. Think Zara with J. Crew, or Aritzia pieces next to designer names in your closet—that's the way you should do it. Danielle also helped me figure out how to dress better for my body type so that I could look sleek rather than…dare I say it… *old!* We've added a lot of tailored blazers, some ballet flats, some great designer purses (I love Chanel), and cute two-piece sets.

Let's not forget how jewelry can age us too. The easiest way to be on the younger side of jewelry looks is to keep up with what's in style. Danielle tells me that right now, the most up-to-date trends are chunky gold earrings, layering necklaces, statement earrings—like hoops or drops, chain necklaces, initial necklaces, and classic pieces like Bulgari watches. You can't go wrong if you stay classic with a little bit of edge. Stay away from pearls and big diamonds. And two or three ear piercings on each ear is good—no need for more than that.

Oh, and I swear by the Stylebook app. It lets you upload pictures of pieces in your closet—clothes, shoes, and accessories—and then you can match items together. It's so helpful to use when packing for a vacation too. When Danielle and I come up with an outfit, I file it into the app so I'll remember. It makes getting ready foolproof. I like to say, have an outfit ready to go for every occasion (while working within your budget, of course) and make sure it fits right (we'll get to the very important topic of tailoring later in this chapter!).

Working with a personal stylist can get expensive, with services usually running you between $100 and $300 an hour. But the really expensive part is this: I keep a credit card on file with Danielle. She'll text me when she sees pieces she thinks I'll like. It's soooo hard to say no to something if I love it! And I seem to love everything she sends me. I'll admit it—I buy way more than I need!

Now I'll turn it over to Danielle.

STYLING
Words from the Wise:
Danielle Klein,
Personal Shopper & Stylist

The first thing I always do with a new client is a closet cleanout, like I did with Sandy. We take inventory of everything a person has, and we work from there. I want to make sure any new pieces we bring in are unique to that person's personal preferences, so we spend time talking about that too.

Once the client's closet is fully cleaned out, I start searching for pieces my clients might like. When I see something, I'll send it to them (I work both in-person in the Los Angeles area and virtually). The client can then decide what they like best from the pieces I've suggested for them. Slowly, we build a closet they love. I also help my clients with any big events they have coming up, like a black-tie or a red-carpet event. I'll come up with that outfit and any accessory options to choose from. They pick what they like the most for those occasions.

Whether my client is in their twenties or their sixties, I like to encourage them to dress tastefully and age-appropriately. We aim to keep classic pieces in their closet, like blazers and ballet flats. You don't need to spend a ton of money to achieve a mix of more expensive timeless pieces with affordable staples. Another trick I tell my clients is this: If you can't afford the St. Laurent piece, get some vintage St. Laurent buttons and switch them onto a Zara piece.

And I always tell my clients to tailor their clothes. You absolutely must have your pieces altered. If you take an expensive designer outfit that's not tailored and compare it to one from Zara that is, the Zara outfit will look better 100 percent of the time.

If you're interested in finding a personal shopper, start by looking into stylists online whose personal style resonates with you. Don't be afraid to try out different stylists, too, until you find the perfect fit. And keep in mind that many stylists also do virtual sessions like I do, so you don't need to necessarily hire someone in your area. Keep your options open! If you find a stylist who understands your vision, you'll be able to easily achieve your style goals.

The Right Fit is "Sew" Crucial

Style isn't just what you wear, it's about how it fits too. This goes beyond finding the right clothes and clothing size for your body. Which brings me to my next topic: tailoring. One of my biggest secret weapons (who am I kidding? I have no secrets!) is my tailor, Elie Paul.

I met Elie when I first moved to Miami Beach—he has a shop here—and it was like the stars aligned. I see Elie more than I see my own family! He's taught me so much about sizing and how to make sure I never, ever look like a sausage in a casing! I bring everything to him, and he takes the outfits I love and turns them into outfits I *LOVE*!! When a piece fits right, it's flattering. It's *on* to the eye. Elie is so special, and he brings an insane level of attention to detail in everything I bring him.

You can tell a fit isn't right when you're drowning in excess fabric or when the seams look like they're going to bust. When that happens, bring it to a tailor! Repeat after me: When in doubt, tailor it out.

TAILORING
Words from the Wise:
Elie Paul, Tailor

I've been tailoring since I was fifteen years old, when I was a kid growing up in Haiti. I came to the U.S. in 1976 and since then I've tailored in New Jersey, Georgia, and now Miami Beach. I do all kinds of jobs for my clients, from minor alterations to complete custom creation, like I often do for Sandy.

I like to refer to Sandy as the "queen of the shop!" We love her here—I've been working with her for years, so I know exactly what she's looking for, and tailor to her needs. Sometimes we'll even transform entire designer pieces into something brand new. We make sure everything fits her perfectly, and that's what I do for all of my clients.

Tailored pieces can elevate a person's style. For this reason, I like to get to know my clients likes and needs so I can create garments that not only fit perfectly but also make them look how they want to look.

I always say, I'm going to die at my sewing machine, and I mean it! I love the work I do more than anything. Find a tailor who feels the same, and you're set for life.

Locks & Loaded:
Prepare to Love Your Hair

Let's move on to hair, shall we? Hair can accomplish the same effect as clothes—it can either age you, or it can reverse-age you. Not to keep bringing up *The Brady Bunch,* but I recently came across a side-by-side picture of Alice, the woman who played the maid in the show. One picture showed her with the hairstyle she wore on the show, super short and mousy brown. The other picture showed her with a photoshopped hairstyle, long and a pretty brown color with highlights. I swear she looked twenty years younger in the photoshopped image!

If you want to look young, not all hairstyles are created equal. Let's start with very short haircuts. I don't mean a sleek bob; I'm talking about the overly severe short haircut. Just like Alice's "before" photo, that hair wasn't helping anyone! You know the style I mean, right? It's so stiff and immobile looking that it could double as a crash helmet. What's worse is combining short hair with, OMG I don't even want to type it…a *perm.* Good God!

Then, there's color. Listen, I respect women who want to age gracefully. But when you go gray, it can age you without a doubt. That salt and pepper look is not reminiscent of youth, that's just a fact. And those young women who intentionally dye their hair gray? Are you leaving the salon and heading to Bingo, or what…?

An excellent hair stylist can easily guide you toward youthful cuts and colors that are right for you based on your natural hair texture and color. They can also help you keep your hair healthy. Because dead, unhealthy hair can look old too.

My trusted hair stylist here in Miami is Kelly Godinez (@kelly_godinez on Instagram). Together, she and I have brought my hair to new lengths! But before we get into that, I want to go on a little detour for a minute to tell you about my hair journey. In my forties I started to notice my hair falling out in clumps. I never had an issue like this with hair loss before and it scared the *bleep* out of me! I turned to wigs for a while, but it didn't put the brakes on my concern. Then I found a dermatologist in New York City, Dr. Joel Kassimir. He took one look at me and knew exactly what was going on: My DHT levels were off.

I wasn't even sure what DHT (dihydrotestosterone) was until I met Dr. Kassimir, but he explained that DHT is produced in the body as a byproduct of testosterone. I didn't tend to think of testosterone and women in the same sentence, but like we talked about earlier, women need it too. But, when our bodies produce too much or too little of it, it can cause our hair follicles to shrink, leading to hair loss. Based on my hair pattern, Dr. Kassimir easily diagnosed it, and then my bloodwork confirmed it. He suggested I take a DHT blocker every day. It took about a few months, but lo and behold, this man was right! My hair started to grow back, and I finally got to bid adieu to my wig.

Another supplement for hair growth that works great is one that my naturopath, Dr. Nadia Musavvir, created called Healthy Hair (it's available through her website www.drmusavvir.com if you're interested). It has biotin, copper, and zinc in it, and unlike most hair supplements that only contain herbs and nutrients that target the impact of androgens on hair, Healthy Hair contains herbs and nutrients that target the impact of both androgens and excess estrogens on the hair follicle.

There are lots of different reasons for thinning hair, but if you're struggling with it, I suggest you see a dermatologist and ask some questions. I know so many women who just slab on some drugstore product that promises hair growth, then get disappointed when it doesn't work. Ask the professional!

Now, back to my beloved hair styling professional, Kelly. Kelly has seen me through that terrible, thin hair phase and wig. Once I had some growth, she added weft extensions for some length and volume, which saved me too. And she's always known the right cut to make me feel good. Here's her expert advice on cuts and extensions.

HAIR CUTS & EXTENSIONS
Words from the Wise:
Kelly Godinez, Hair Stylist

The first step to finding a hairstyle that works for you, and helps you look younger, is to find a hair stylist who's up to date with trends. Social media can be helpful for finding the right stylist, as it essentially shows you a portfolio of that person's work.

I think a sleek bob is a great choice for everyone—something blunt and right above the shoulder. It makes a person look elegant and chic. Years ago, it was in style to do an angled bob, where the back of the hair was slightly shorter than the front, but it's now outdated. And an outdated hairstyle will make you look older. If you're not into the bob and would rather keep your hair longer, I recommend nipple-length, with face framing layers in the front. Very long hair will make you look older as you age, too, so that mid-to-long length is a great spot for you to be.

As my clients age, their biggest concern is often volume. As we age, our hair will naturally get thinner, and it can be made worse with stress, major sicknesses, and even post surgeries. Extensions are a great option to help with volume. If you're considering extensions, the most important thing is to find the right stylist and to do a consultation. During the consultation, the stylist should go over all of your options (there are various type of extensions) and help determine what the right kind is for you, your hair type, and your goals. The right stylist won't just sell you the type of extensions they know how to do—they should be honest.

Clip-in extensions are a good option for someone who is interested in fuller hair for events, or someone who doesn't have the budget to come in every three months to get the extensions professionally redone. Clip ins are very easy to use—anyone can do it at home. Tape-in extensions are another option, as well as the popular weft extensions, which can be either sewn or glued in. Fusion or bonded extensions are a more permanent solution, and are individually attached. Then, there are micro-link extensions, and they use tiny beads to secure the extension strand to the client's real hair. For any professionally installed extensions, I recommend my clients with extensions come in every four weeks to move up the extensions, and once every three months to remove everything and put them back in.

If your hair is very thin, extensions might not be a good option, as you might risk more hair loss. You might be better off with a wig.

Keeping your hair looking good means keeping it healthy too. I tell my clients to avoid blow drying their hair more than two times a week, and always use a heat protectant before blow drying or using other hot tools. I recommend only shampooing two to three times a week, depending on hair texture.

Your hair is at its weakest when it's wet, so be careful when brushing wet hair, and start from the ends and work up to the root as you brush. Avoid pulling your hair into a bun when it's wet—tugging it back will easily lead to breakage. Even if it's dry, don't keep your hair in a tight bun all week. Let your hair down!

Sleek buns look gorgeous, but can hurt your hair too. Instead of wrapping the sleek bun up in a scrunchie, do a ponytail instead and use bobby pins to pin up the bun. Wrapping your hair tightly into a bun with a scrunchie can cause breakage, and the bobby pins will be easier on the hair.

I recommend clean, eco-friendly hair products. I love the TRUSS brand. Your hair will thank you for using a great shampoo and conditioner. Always read the ingredients! Think of it this way: You spend the money on your hair at the hair salon to make sure it looks great—why not spend the extra dollars to keep it up day-to-day?

Having a great hairstyle and boosting up that volume are so important, but so is hair color. I've been getting my hair dyed by master colorist Erica Quince (@ericaquincecolors on Instagram), the co-owner of House of Mane in Miami (www.houseofmane.com). Much like my other experts, Erica is a freakin' genius. My natural hair color is a dark blonde, but the vibrant blonde she's been able to achieve is stunning. She's also taught me a ton about keeping my dyed hair healthy.

HAIR COLOR
Words from the Wise:
Erica Quince, Hair Colorist

I've been in the business for over twelve years, and during that time, I've been lucky enough to help so many clients get the confidence boost they're looking for from a great hair color. I've had clients literally cry when we've brought their hair back to life. Moments like that make me happy to do what I do. For me, it's not just about making money; it's about bringing out the beauty in everyone and making them feel their best. I always prioritize the health of my clients' hair—there's really nothing more important than that. Your hair is only going to look good if it's healthy, that's just a fact.

Choosing the right person to trust with your hair is fundamental. They'll be able to help you get a great color while keeping your hair healthy. When clients ask me to help them figure out the right hair color for them, I guide them toward finding a color that complements their skin tone and enhances their features. We always recommend against our brunettes who want to go blonde too quickly. It can absolutely kill the hair. For Sandy, we did a gradual transition to blonde highlights, which helped maintain the health of her hair.

Having amazing hair isn't only about your visits to the salon; it's also about how you treat your hair every day. I tell my clients that proper care and maintenance on a daily basis will make so much of a difference. For example, many people tend to over-wash their hair, and that can strip their hair of essential oils. I recommend against washing every day for that very reason. It's also a good idea to get a filter for your showerhead. And it's important to remember how fragile wet hair is—it needs to be handled gently to prevent breakage, so no tight buns when your hair is wet.

I recommend investing in quality hair products to care for your hair at home. A product line I like a lot is K18 Hair. It's important to change products every so often—just like you would with skincare products—so that your hair doesn't get used to them. A lot of people also overlook scalp health. I recommend regular scalp treatments that can help hair growth, texture, and overall hair health.

Of course, take caution with at home hair dyes! Leave the color corrections to the professionals; DIY disasters can be costly when you have to go to professionals to fix it anyway (and DIY jobs can be very damaging). There's a reason we spend years honing our skills as colorists. It's not just about slapping on color or applying treatments—it's about knowing how different hair types will react and tailoring the right approach. Be sure to look for a trusted professional who understands the complexities of hair chemistry.

I want to make sure I'm also meeting the client's unique needs and preferences. It should be a collaborative process. I want my clients to trust me, and whoever your colorist is should feel the same.

Here is the customized approach we've come up with for Sandy:

- I do a half head of highlights and use a lightener (bleach), making sure to not overlap the pieces that have already been highlighted.
- In between the foils I paint the gray hair with a semi-permanent color.

- I do a combination of baby light and heavier weave to have a different variation of blonde and to create dimension.
- I keep the foils in until the hair is a buttery tone and then rinse the sections as they're ready.
- I'll then shampoo and do a root smudge so there isn't a line of color, and it blends better and allows the hair to grow out nicely.
- The last step is an all-over gloss, which blends the hair together nicely and adds shine.
- The goal throughout the whole process is to avoid damage.

Lhonette Bernard Charles (@lhonettehair on Instagram) is another hair colorist who's very popular in Miami. She is the co-owner of Studio Raūpo (@studio.raupo on Instagram). She is known for keeping hair colors looking vibrant, and importantly, for keeping her clients' hair very healthy. Here's the protocol Lhonette follows.

HAIR COLOR
Words from the Wise:
Lhonette Bernard Charles, Hair Colorist

For my clients who dye their hair lighter, I do not allow them to color it more than once every five to six months. My goal is to keep my clients' hair healthy, and overprocessed hair is just the opposite of that. If their natural hair is a lot darker and they're concerned about roots, I have them come in every two to three months to do a semi-permanent gloss for their roots. This helps blend the color and the quality of their hair won't be affected. That semi-permanent gloss will last about twenty washes.

Even if a client insists on full highlights every three months, I'll turn them away. It just isn't healthy, and the way I see it, my clients' hair speaks for me. When they're walking down the street, it's an advertisement for my work. If their hair is fried and ruined, what would that say about my work? I want them to be happy and I want my existing clients—and my new clients—to trust me. Beware of a colorist who tells you you need to come back every three months when there's bleach involved. You're only going to be spending more while ruining the quality of your hair.

Brushing Up on Makeup

In Chapter 3 we talked about permanent makeup options, but what about daily makeup application? Nothing brings your whole look together like gorgeous makeup. I know what some of you reading this will think: *Ugh, Sandy! But I'm awful at doing my own makeup!*

Trust me, it's easier than you think, especially if you keep it simple. Makeup artist Angelique Cecchetti (@makeupangelique on Instagram and portfolio at www.AngeliqueCecchetti.myportfolio.com) has taught me everything there is to know about using makeup to age backward. She knows all the best techniques and products to enhance a person's features and leave them looking refreshed and revitalized. She's also created different face charts for me to follow so I know exactly what to use for day and night. (Naturally, we go lighter for day, darker for night.)

Here's Angelique's advice for achieving a youthful look with makeup application.

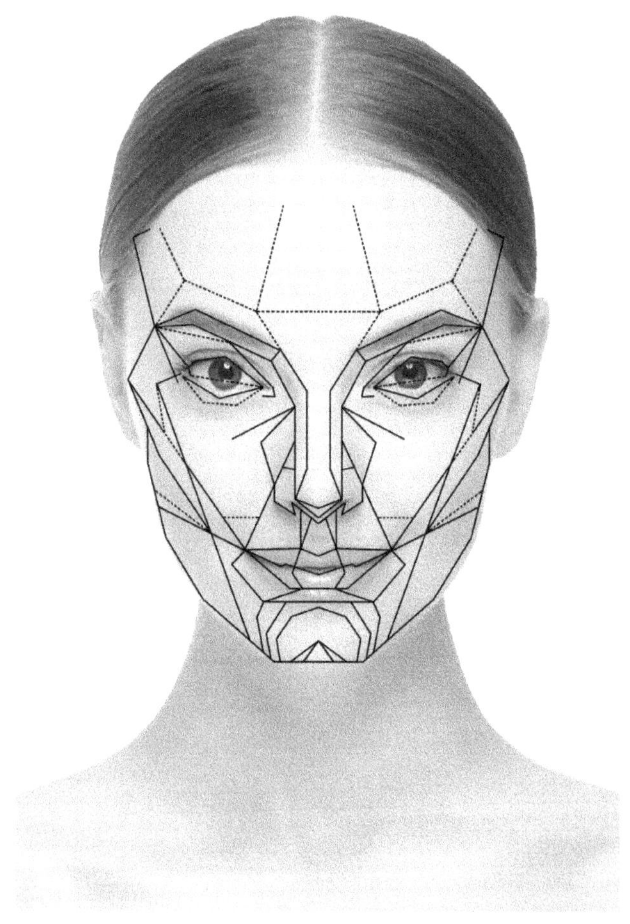

MAKEUP APPLICATION
Words from the Wise:
Angelique Cecchetti,
Professional Makeup Artist

It's always important to start with skincare—it's the key to glowy skin. Hydrated skin appears plumper and more youthful. Also, without skincare, makeup won't hold the same way (you'll notice the makeup will look separated and patchy). You want to make sure the makeup will go on evenly and that it stays put. Think of your skincare routine as creating a smooth canvas for your makeup.

I use what's called a "face chart" in my make-up lessons with the clients. It's a makeup drawing that shows exactly what I've taught the client in our makeup session, and I list all of the products I used, the order of how to apply them, and I include other notes to help them easily remember the steps.

For my clients who are trying to achieve a young-er look, I first suggest liquid instead of compact when it comes to what's applied to the skin. Liquid will always be easier to apply and offers a stretching texture compared to a compact foundation, con-cealer, or compact powder.

I also recommend matte eyeshadow instead of anything shiny, as matte finishing blurs the lines on the eyelid, and anything glittery or shimmery amplifies those lines. In terms of colors, I suggest a bronzy eye look (a mix of earthy tones, like brown, beige, yellow, and copper). You can't go wrong with those shades—it doesn't matter your eye color or the skin color … it always works. Use a light color on the inner corner of the eye and a darker color on the outer corner, then blend them together with a bronzing powder and a small brush (like Mac's brush #217) in the crease to break any lines. Stay away from purple and burgundy eyeshadows (and everything with red) if you have dark circles; they will only accentuate them and give you a tired look.

Make sure to give some love to your eyebrows. It can be an eyebrow pencil or eyebrow mascara—either way it will help lift up your eyes. Use a color corrector under your eyes if you have dark circles as that will help to neutralize the shadow of the dark circle. It will also prevent you from having to use too much concealer (we don't like a lot of texture under the eyes, so this helps reduce the amount of product there).

My key to a fresh look is blush. I'm personally a big blush lover and I think there's no such thing as too much. Find your perfect pink tone and stick with it daily—there's nothing bad about showing your cheekbones!

To finish, add lip liner, as it really helps to redefine the lips. It's the best trick to overline, which gives the effects of full and plump lips, and it also prevents lipstick bleeding.

I don't believe in one specific brand across the board. I have my favorite products in a few different brands, but that doesn't mean they are good for everyone. Instead of focusing on brands, I would just say that what you need to achieve a good makeup look are good brushes. Without the right brushes, you cannot expect to have a professional result. You can have the best makeup products, but without good brushes, your application will be really limited.

For a daytime look, I avoid anything heavy. I believe less is more for day. Makeup moves throughout the day, so a look that is great when you leave home can turn very unflattering two hours later. I would rather see real skin with a few imperfections than heavy textures that age you. There is nothing less chic than a dirty makeup look. A fresh face is so much nicer and shows you're taking care of your looks without trying to hide yourself under pounds of makeup.

For those interested in having a professional makeup artist do your look for you, costs can vary from about $150 if booked through something like a glam squad app (yes, that exists!) to $500 and up if booked through an agency. Those prices are for a full glam makeup look.

No Man Hands!

In my opinion, nothing looks as *"WTF!"* as a woman's hands when her fingernails are chewed down, bare, or look like she's been digging in the dirt for a year. Every time I see that, I cringe. Those are what I like to call *man hands*. Hands are so, so easy (and affordable) to take care of…why neglect them?

It's pretty easy to avoid getting man hands in the first place. For example, next time you're heading out to work on your garden, wear freakin' gloves. But what if you have a job that requires you to use your hands a lot? Even then, there's basic maintenance that you can do. Start by cleaning that dirt out from underneath those nails, then clip and file them, and throw on a coat of clear nail polish. And if that sounds like too much maintenance, keep in mind that a regular manicure only costs about $20 at most salons.

There's a definite *je ne sais quoi* about a woman with well-manicured nails! It just looks so much nicer. Now, I'm not saying that you need long nails, bold patterns, or bright colors that pop. Even the most minimalistic look will do the trick. Manicured hands can pull an entire look together. But man hands DO NOT! Unless you're going for a lumberjack look, that is.

And if you need further motivation to get into the salon, how about the fact that it's also therapeutic! If you're anything like me, it'll give you a little confidence boost. My nail tech is Haya Amer (@purenailsstudio on Instagram) and I go at least once every other week to keep my nails looking flawless.

NAILS
Words from the Wise:
Haya Amer, Nail Technician

I've seen some rough hands come through the salon. As Sandy says, we're not a fan of "man hands," so I clean those hands up and make them look like lady hands again. Sometimes it's someone who just doesn't have enough time for upkeep and there's way too much growth, making the nails look really…troubled! I've even seen people come in with black fungus on their nails. So nasty!

I recommend gel polish to my clients because it lasts, but if they don't want to do that, even a manicure and clean up does the trick. There's a big trend right now with natural nails—either unpainted or using natural nail polish, and that's great too, as long as the dirt is out from under the nails and those cuticles are trimmed down. Having your nails done is also an excellent form of self-care.

There's been a lot of talk lately about whether the lights that are used to dry UV gel nail polish at the salon are harmful to you, and I assure you, they're not. Your hands get more UV rays from fifteen seconds of sitting on the steering wheel on a sunny day than they do under the UV lights at the nail salon dryer.

Growing strong and healthy nails doesn't have to be this huge mystery, or done with fake nail extensions! In fact, it's all about understanding how what you eat affects your nail growth and strength. If you find that your nails are constantly looking dry and cracked, don't forget the importance of taking care of them from the inside out. Eating a balanced diet with the right vitamins is essential for growing your nails out naturally.

Vitamin A is key for healthy nail growth. You can get it from dairy, leafy greens, eggs, and carrots. Vitamin B is another great nail strengthening vitamin. It can be found in whole grains, beans, eggs, fish, and more. Biotin is a B vitamin that helps your body convert food into energy and plays an important role in nail growth and strength! Vitamin C is also key for nail health, and can be found in citrus fruits, peppers, strawberries and other fruits and vegetables.

It's also important to get enough iron and calcium, which are essential for healthy nails. You can find iron in red meat, poultry, fish, beans, and dark leafy greens. Calcium is found in dairy, dark leafy greens, and fortified cereals and juices. Calcium is essential for forming strong nails and helps to protect them from breakage.

Health is important, and you can see it in the health of your nails. Eating the right foods with the right vitamins and minerals is essential for strong, healthy nails. With the right diet and vitamins, you can grow your nails out naturally and have the healthy nails you've always dreamed of.

If you look the part of a young woman, it'll help you feel like one too. And when you feel good about your clothes, hair, makeup, and nails, your confidence will shoot through the roof. People will be turning their heads thinking, *Hey, that young lady looks great!* The world is your runway!

CHAPTER ELEVEN

A DIET AND WORKOUT THAT WORKS

Let me give it to you plain and simple: The best diet and workout routine for women over forty is calorie counting, weightlifting, and walking forty-five minutes a day (you want a low impact cardio routine to prevent injuries). No frills at all. Plus, it's easy to do (and stick to!) when you know what you're doing.

I'll start with diets. Back in Chapter 6, I wrote about most women's desire to be thin, and I listed some fad diets too many of us have tried. The thing about fad diets is…they don't work! Like, ever. You might lose a few pounds, but most of that weight loss isn't sustainable because the diet isn't sustainable.

Fad Diets Are Doomed to Fail (And Not Just Because You're Hangry)

Fad diets take a toll on our bodies. They keep us in starvation mode. They have us eating cabbage soup, or consuming only raw foods, or spooning mashed-up baby food out of those little jars (like, WTF!). I even heard that back in the 1920s, there was something called the "cigarette diet"—how disgusting. (I've mentioned this previously, but smoking is the worst thing you can do to your body. It ages your face, yes, but it also leaves your lungs looking like the inside of a filthy ashtray. Eww!)

It's a false belief that crash diets rev up your metabolism, when in fact, they do just the opposite. You're basically depriving your body of the nutrients and calories it needs. A fad diet tricks your metabolism into thinking it's in starvation mode, which causes it to slow down and hold on for dear life to every calorie you consume. Not to mention, it leaves us super pissed and hangry all the time. Sure, you may shed a few pounds in the process, but at what cost—your sanity?

So, your metabolism is shot, *and* your mood is shot. Then, when you start eating regularly again—or worse, binge-eating an entire box of donuts because you're so deprived—BOOM! The number on the scale will jump right back up. What a waste of time!

Don't even get me started on how many people rely on Ozempic for weight loss without even attempting a proper diet and exercise routine first! When it comes to weight loss, Ozempic is for people with obesity—not someone who wants to lose ten pounds. There is so little research as of right now on the long-term effects of Ozempic and similar drugs when used for weight loss and I'm shocked at how many people aren't scared of that fact. Not to mention the changes Ozempic makes to a person's face! Heard of Ozempic face? Or Ozempic butt? Look it up! Yikes.

The Simple Art of Counting Calories

If you want to lose weight, the best way to do it is to count calories. (As a general rule of thumb, I also drink plenty of water throughout the day, and get eight hours of sleep a night—both are so important.) Yeah, calorie counting is not as chic as a juice cleanse or whatever the latest superfood diet is from the Amazon rainforest, but hey, it works. The truth is, calorie counting is the only way to stay consistent with your diet. It's just math. Every time you eat something, tally up the calories consumed. Now, I'm by no means recommending you spend all your daily calories on junk food—you should be mindful to mix in the right nutrients. (But don't deprive yourself of a treat if you want it.)

I started counting calories during the COVID-19 pandemic and found it easy to do, especially if you use a free app like MyFitnessPal. The app lets you quickly search the foods and ingredients you've consumed that day and totals your calorie intake for you. (You can also use the app to scan barcodes from food labels, too, so it's foolproof.)

I happen to be a vegetarian, so I tend to eat a lot of the same foods every day. I quickly learned the calorie count of the foods I eat. Now I don't even need the app anymore! I can add the calories in my head. Usually, I aim for 1,200 calories per day. And I don't subtract the calories I burn during my workouts. I will, however, add 200 more calories and carbs on leg day—specifically I'll add 40 percent protein, 40 percent carbs and 20 percent fat. (Keep in mind, building muscles often adds numbers to the scale—but who cares about the number if you're looking and feeling fit? In a year I gained seven and a half pounds from building muscle, but that number doesn't bother me because my hard work resulted in me now only having thirteen percent body fat.) Please consult with a nutritionist about what's right for you.

While counting calories, I do try to keep in mind this graphic I've seen that shows you are what you eat. For this reason, I try my best to keep sugar out of my diet because it plays a big role in inflammation, which is of course, some-thing we all want to avoid at all costs (remember, we hate *puff!*). You'll notice in this graphic that dairy, gluten, and wine take a toll on our faces as well. Overconsumption can have real effects.

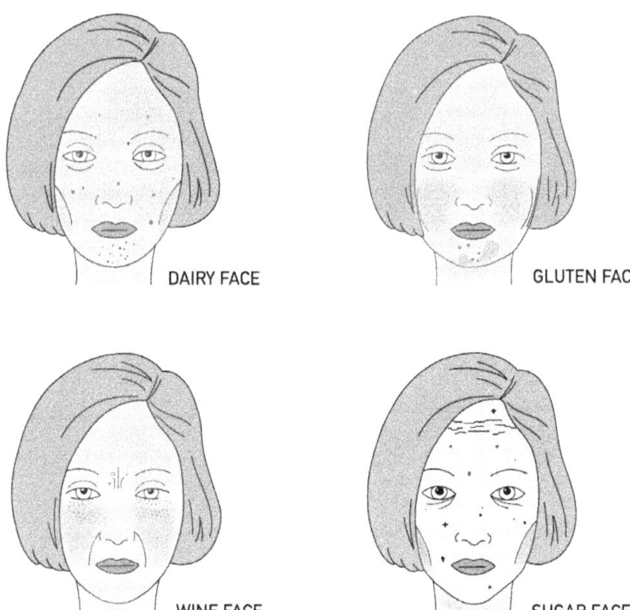

I'm not saying I never eat sugar, dairy, or gluten (I never have wine, though)—if I'm craving something delicious, like a warm, gooey chocolate chip cookie right out of the oven that's calllllling my name (can you tell that's a weak spot for me?), I won't deny myself. But I try not to eat a ton of it, if possible. So, if you're at a party or an event and you crave a treat, don't deny yourself. If you try to fully eliminate certain foods you love, you could be likely to binge on them later. Let's face it, we're all human.

My Hot Take:
Say "No" to Alcohol!

Now, this is something I feel very passionate about: Alcohol is bad for you! That's why I never drink it. In the very few instances when I'm out somewhere and I order a drink with dinner (*very rare!!*), I'll pretend to take a couple of sips. I understand this may be a very hot take—I know women out there love their wine specifically—but hear me out. The sobering reality (pun intended) is that alcohol is full of toxins. As we age, our metabolism naturally starts to slow down, which means those toxins we drink are sticking around longer in our system. Your liver goes into overdrive too, processing the alcohol and toxins more slowly as you age.

Our bodies also hold onto less water as we get older. Yes, that means even if you're drinking endless refills in your beloved Stanley cup all day. Decreased water combined with any amount of booze means a higher blood alcohol concentration. If you've noticed that you get tipsy from drinking a bit of alcohol far more easily than you did in your twenties, it's not your imagination— it's biology!

No wonder hangovers become so horrible with age! The morning after drinking is like a horror movie and you're the lead character. It's the body saying, "Remember when we used to be able to bounce back from this? Good times, good times…"

Don't get me wrong, it's not like I *never* drank. I used to love social drinking. Years ago, it didn't affect me like it does now (and it makes a lot of sense given what we just talked about). These days, I just don't want to feel like crap though. I'm doing everything else to make myself feel good, why ruin it with alcohol? When I stopped drinking, I had more energy, had less anxiety (WOO!), and was a lot less irritable. I loved never having a foggy brain the entire next day after a social event. While friends were complaining of headaches and curled up in a ball next to a Gatorade, I was at the gym!

Plus, if the goal is to feel young, booze just isn't the way to do it. I came across a 2022 study from the publication *Nature* that stuck with me. It found that people who were fifty years old and had consumed one beer or one glass of wine per day for the previous month had brain cells that appeared two years older (!!) than those who'd only had half that amount. This blew my mind! They didn't report on how this compared to non-drinkers, but I can only imagine what those results would show.

My close friend Veida Horn (@veidasadridesign on Instagram) has spent years researching the negative effects of alcohol, especially wine, on our bodies. Here's her stance on it.

ALCOHOL
Words from the Wise:
Veida Horn

These days, people tend to glorify wine, especially women. For example, you often hear moms say they "need" a glass of wine after a day of taking care of the kids. My take is—if you need wine to raise children—that's not a good thing.

Even women without children tend to consume wine as a way of self-care. Or they've read a study once that said a glass of red wine a night is good for you. So, they drink for their health. But, in reality, daily wine consumption does not equal improved health—it simply doesn't. There are certainly compounds in wine that have benefits, but to reap them, you'd have to drink more wine than your body could ever process.

I won't lie, there was a time during the pandemic when I was doing this too. But one day I woke up and noticed how all-around bad my body felt. Now I don't drink at home anymore, because I want to prioritize my well-being. Alcohol ages us, and like Sandy, I want to do the reverse.

American wines have a ton of additives, sugar, and pesticides. If you are going to drink wine, pay attention to where it comes from and how it's produced. Prioritize quality over price. Keep in mind that just because a bottle of wine is expensive doesn't mean it won't give you a hangover. And be mindful of certain brands' misleading marketing claims.

I understand the temptation to drink can be there. Socializing often goes hand-in-hand with alcohol consumption. I won't say I never have a drink when I'm socializing, but that habit of having a glass of wine every night at home is just not good. To the best of your ability, try to prioritize yourself over social pressures to drink.

If you're someone who likes having a drink during dinner at a restaurant, there are lots of places that have great mocktail menus with nonalcoholic options. If you do want a drink, stick to a maximum of three drinks. I also recommend against sugary mixers that can add lots of unnecessary calories. Moderation is important—as is being mindful.

What if you decide to indulge, you drink too much, and that inevitable hangover hits? Don't turn to greasy food! Instead, opt for a smoothie packed with protein, berries, and yogurt. Rehydrate and engage in some physical activity. It will help with the physical hangover, plus it will also help fight any anxiety that might creep up that day (they don't call them the "scaries" for nothing!).

As I was wrapping up writing this book, both Veida and my husband, Dave, decided to stop drinking alcohol completely, and they've said it has made such a huge difference in their bodies in just sixty days. Both of them have eczema and, in addition to feeling better overall from eliminating alcohol, their eczema has also cleared up. If you need yet another reason to avoid drinking, there you go!

Dumbbells & Determination

There is only one answer for how to keep things toned and tight with exercise as you age… and that's weight training. During the Covid pandemic, I went from *soft* to *toned* by lifting weights with my personal trainer, Vanessa Reggiardo (again, she's @vanereggia_fit on Instagram). I came out of quarantine looking pretty much the opposite of everyone else; where most people gained weight from overeating, drinking too much, and staying inactive, I was lifted and lighter! My inflammation was completely gone, and I was ten pounds slimmer. I looked and felt the best I had in years. And my skin wasn't sagging all over my body like many other women in their fifties.

The trick to maintaining that muscle tone is staying consistent. That's the part people find the most difficult. But Vanessa and I make training fun! And that's what keeps me coming back to the gym six days a week. Honestly, I don't even dread it. (And I've definitely dreaded certain workouts in the past—like running…*ick!*)

Okay, okay...I know you might be thinking, "Well, what about cardio? Cardio is important!" And I don't necessarily disagree. But cardio shouldn't be your sole source of exercise if you want to keep your body tight and fight the otherwise inevitable sag. Cardio is important for the heart but not to lose weight. Cardio doesn't help you lose weight. Diet and weights help you lose weight. Weightlifting is where the real magic comes in. I know people who love hot yoga and Pilates, who run half marathons and everything in between, and I won't discredit those people or their results. But let's say you're trying to bid farewell to cellulite, for example. Have you ever seen a muscular person with cellulite? I bet not, right? That's because the more muscle you build, the less cellulite you'll have. Weightlifting also helps our bone health by increasing bone density, which is important as you age.

Oh! And weight training builds muscle mass, which boosts your metabolism, even at rest. This means you're burning calories long after your workout session ends. For every pound of muscle you add, you burn an extra fifty calories a day, even while you're resting. It's something to think about.

A common misconception is that lifting weights will make you *bigger.* **Weights don't make you bigger, food does!** (I learned that saying from Vanessa, and it's so true.) Weight training doesn't mean you need to prepare to become the next contender for the World's Strongest Woman, puffing and grunting under a barbell heavy enough to squash a small car! It's more about getting your body lean and mean and amping up your metabolism.

I highly recommend personal training, though it can get expensive, depending on where you are and who you go to. I've seen costs as low as $40 an hour and as high as $400+ an hour.

I'll let Vanessa tell you about the routine she and I practice six days a week. It's not scary or impossible, I promise. In a perfect world, we like to do one hour of weight training and then one hour of lymphatic work…if I'm not late!

WEIGHT TRAINING
Words from the Wise:
Vanessa Reggiardo, Personal Trainer

Since Sandy is a vegetarian, she needs to make sure she's getting enough protein in her diet so that she can build muscle. By the time she's working out in the morning, she's already consumed seventy grams of protein, which is in the range she needs to build muscle. Getting the right amount of protein is often something people forget, but it's really important.

Sandy and I weight train six days per week. We start with five minutes of rowing to get warmed up. Then, we alternate chest/back/shoulders twice a week, legs twice a week, arms twice a week, and core strengthening twice a week. We do a lot of compound work due to the fact that several muscle groups collaborate to perform movement. This includes bench presses, deadlifts, squats and pull ups. Those are the best fat loss exercises. You read that right. They drop fat, build muscle, and get you ripped.

I like to say, if it doesn't hurt, it doesn't work! The best workouts will leave you feeling sore. But even though the weight training might hurt, the results are always worth it. Plus, we keep it fun.

One thing I always remind my clients of is the importance of consistency with weight training. If a client is going on vacation, I tell them they need to get into the gym at their hotel if they don't want to lose the muscle they've built. It only takes two weeks of being off a weightlifting routine before muscle mass starts to decrease. All of that hard work will have been for nothing!

Fascia-nating Insight into the Body

Another important part of my morning with Vanessa is our lymphatic work, which I mentioned quickly way back in the Introduction. This helps with depuffing, and I've seen it help totally diminish my cellulite, too! I have literally *no* cellulite now after using this combination of weightlifting, the right supplements, and regular lymphatic work.

After my workout, we go right into this, and we start by targeting my body's fascia. Fascia is the connective tissue that surrounds the body's muscles, bones, and organs. When pressure is applied to the fascia in strategic ways, it helps me debloat. It's crazy how much of a change I've noticed with bloat in my entire body from using a tool called the FasciaBlaster on my legs to get that fluid moving. (The tool is fairly cheap too. You can find it online for about $100.)

This is what Vanessa has to say about lymphatic drainage and what, exactly, the FasciaBlaster is.

LYMPHATIC DRAINAGE
Words from the Wise:
Vanessa Reggiardo, Personal Trainer

During the pandemic, Sandy and I got into the routine of doing a one-hour workout in the morning and then stretching for an hour later in the afternoon. During our stretching sessions, I noticed Sandy was retaining some water in her legs. I suggested we use a FasciaBlaster to massage her legs and help with her circulation. The FasciaBlaster is a tool created by a woman named

Ashley Black; the tool targets the—you guessed it—fascia in our bodies, which is the connective tissue we have underneath the skin that surrounds our muscles and organs. The FasciaBlaster almost looks like a pizza roller with plastic claws. We started noticing results right away with how Sandy looked and felt. Even though we weren't using the tool on her face, we noticed a lot of decreased water retention there, since her circulation had now improved.

Now we use the tool on Sandy six days a week. After our workout, two times a week we'll do a quick foot scraping (which is just as it sounds) and have Sandy moisturize her feet with socks on. Then we move on to our everyday routine: She'll use her LED mask for ten minutes while I then use the FasciaBlaster on her legs. I massage the front and back parts of her legs (we rotate front and back from day to day) and use the tool on each leg for ten minutes with repeated, gentle upward strokes. We like to use a product called Lipo Cream on her legs while I'm doing this. It works really well at preventing water retention and fighting inflammation, and it's helped get rid of any cellulite she had before. I'd recommend anyone who retains a lot of water to add the FasciaBlaster to their daily routine. You'll be shocked at how different things look very quickly. After that, I use a dry brush on her legs, brushing upward with that as well for ten minutes on each leg.

We also spend time on her face, starting with the FaceGym Multi-Sculpt High-Performance Contouring tool, which we use just like a Gua Sha to depuff her face. Again, we use upward strokes with this tool. We also use a microcurrent device on her face and then a microneedling comb for several minutes. We use the microneedling tool on her stomach for a few minutes too. Finally, we use a self-tanner to round out our morning, and Sandy likes the Tan-Luxe The Gradual Illuminating Tanning Lotion (to avoid looking orange we use only a little) and/or the Hydraboost Gradual Tan Body Butter.

Finding Some Relief

So, as you can tell, my mornings with Vanessa are fun! She and I have become very close friends given how much time we spend together and, of course, how wonderful she is! Everything all came together for me body-wise when we got into this routine. Before all of this though, believe it or not, I was barely able to *stand* let alone lift weights. I'd been in a couple of really bad accidents and the pain I was experiencing in my back and legs was terrible. It was hard to even sit and stand back up! I felt a million years old, and as you can imagine, I HATED IT!

Then I went to Dr. Abhinav Gautam, who co-founded Vitruvia medical center (www.vitruvia.co), here in Miami Beach (he also has a New York City location). Through a treatment he invented called RELIEF, he was able to get me back on my feet. His treatment transformed my life—no exaggeration. It turned out the unbearable pain I was experiencing was being caused by a buildup of scar tissue and nerve damage. He used an ultrasound machine to break up the scar tissue (and in turn help the nerve damage)—it was like watching a video game on the screen as he was doing it.

I'll let Dr. Gautam tell you about what he does, because it's amazing, and can get anyone back on their feet and back to an active and healthy lifestyle and feeling young again.

RELIEF TREATMENT
Words from the Wise:
Dr. Abhinav Gautam,
Vitruvia Co-Founder

With something like back pain, it's so poorly treated by conventional medicine. Often, they'll use X-rays and MRIs to try to see what's going on and then the first step for treatment is a steroid injection, which offers a temporary Band-Aid to the situation. Then the patient is referred to surgery. But the pain isn't always coming from in and around the spinal cord. It's often caused by problems with the fascia—the connective tissue that surrounds the body's muscles, bones, and organs—being too stiff and rigid. In those cases, surgery isn't even the right answer.

In Sandy's case, she was experiencing a lot of pain caused by a buildup of scar tissue and nerve damage due to the car accidents she'd been in. Anytime there's an injury and internal swelling, it can distort the normal scar tissue and the nerves can fuse with the skin, which is what Sandy was experiencing. The nerves were severely compromised, her fascia that was scarred, and there was muscle that had been damaged. Basically, her muscles were stuck in the wrong configurations, and that was the root cause of these problems. With RELIEF, we were able to remodel and reconstruct the soft tissue, and she bounced back with no problems. It's now five years later, and none of that pain has returned.

We use RELIEF to do scar mapping on our patients by first using a high-frequency ultrasound. We then use the ultrasound to separate the tissue. This is done by recreating a fetal microenvironment in affected areas—meaning it tricks the body into thinking it's healing as it did in the womb. Basically what it's doing is stimulating the body's natural regenerative capabilities, breaking up that scar tissue and lessening inflammation.

The treatment is minimally invasive, is done under local anesthesia, takes only about thirty to sixty minutes, and there is no downtime. RELIEF can be used many places on the body: Back, neck, legs, arms, hands, feet, shoulders, hips…you name it.

Now, a few years after this treatment, I can't imagine what my life would be like if I hadn't done it. I love the gym and feel so good about the progress I've made, and I really could not have done it if I was in that amount of pain. I feel great all around, and I recently found something to add to my routine that took me to a whole new level at the gym…and that was bodywork.

You Can Reach Peak Athleticism through Bodywork

I am in the best shape I've ever been because of calorie counting and weight training. But it's also because I've started to do bodywork. Bodywork is a lot like massage—it's a physical manipulation of the body to improve health and well-being. A professional bodywork specialist can stretch and adjust your body in ways that help it function at its best.

It includes hands-on techniques like massage and stretching. But it's different from a regular ol' massage. Massages mainly focus on manipulating muscles and soft tissues to promote relaxation and relieve tension. When you get a massage, they tend to focus on spots you have discomfort in to get circulation going and get rid of any muscle stiffness.

But bodywork is far more, let's say, *comprehensive*. It does all the things that massage can do, but also takes your body's entire overall structure and alignment into consideration. Attention to fascia is important with massage, but *super important* with bodywork. Bodywork techniques specifically target the fascia, and this helps achieve a ton of lengthening in the body and increased flexibility.

I found the best of the best here in Miami—Juancarlos Muguercia (we all call him Swammy—you can find him on Instagram @dr.fascia)—and he stretches me for forty-five minutes twice a week before I go to the gym. I'm longer and leaner, and I've gotten stronger too. On average, the cost of working with a bodywork therapist seems to be between $75 and $150 an hour, money *well* spent!

BODYWORK

Words from the Wise:
Juancarlos Muguercia (AKA "Swammy")

Bodywork tends to get overlooked because not many people understand what it is. When we do bodywork, we focus on the body's fascia, the connective tissue that holds our muscles together. Think of fascia as the wetsuit of the body. It provides structure and support to muscles and organs. During a bodywork session, we'll use our hands to massage the fascia in order to create space within the body, leading to improved posture, circulation, and even a more youthful appearance. So, while a traditional massage focuses on muscle manipulation, body work targets the fascia, which results in more profound and long-lasting changes to the body's structure.

Bodywork focuses on relieving tension, restoring alignment, and optimizing movement patterns. It's about making space. Think of it this way: When you have unreleased stress in the body, your arms and legs tense up, and they become shorter. By using bodywork, stretching with active resistance and massaging the connective tissue, you're relieving that stress and lengthening limbs.

If someone does bodywork consistently—ideally at least once a week—they can notice significant improvements in their posture and overall strength. It can really serve as a missing piece of the puzzle for people on a fitness and wellness journey. I've seen bodywork help everyone from a person with Parkinson's disease, to a paraplegic, to the world's top athletes. Tom Brady is a great example of someone who's used bodywork and has seen remarkable results from doing so consistently. He's known for his age-defying abilities well into his forties.

I approach bodywork by first getting to understand the client's specific needs, as well as any tension patterns, traumas, or injuries they've had over time. We then focus on alleviating any physical discomfort they have. One of the key principles of bodywork is customization. Each session is tailored to that individual's needs and goals, whether it's addressing chronic pain, improving athletic performance, or enhancing overall well-being. We can release tight hamstrings, correct posture imbalances, and so much more.

It's never too early (or too late) to start body-work. I'm a firm believer that bodywork should start young. In terms of education, I think that just as we teach kids the importance of proper nutrition and exercise, schools should teach lessons on posture, alignment, and body awareness. This way we have healthier, more resilient adults.

Bodywork is anti-aging. With better alignment and better circulation, you'll simply look better and feel younger.

With all these things working in my favor, I feel more confident in my body than ever before—and yes, I'm looking at you too, thirty-year-old Sandy! I'm somehow more confident than you were!

I'm working harder now than I ever have be-fore, and I *feel* great! That's what matters. Real-ly, it's not about fitting into a certain size jeans, or sporting a six pack, or having zero cellulite (though I do love that part, I'm not going to lie!). It's about feeling good in your own skin. It's about being aware of what you're putting into your body and how much. And it's about doing activities you love. If the idea of a treadmill makes you cringe, don't use that as your main form of exercise! Do what you like to feel strong, vibrant, and freaking amazing.

CONCLUSION

GOODBYE FOR NOW, BUT NOT FOREVER!

Congratulations! You've done it! You've been inside my brain! (I told you I have no secrets. I like to say, no one could ever blackmail me, because I tell my secrets to everyone.) You now know nearly everything about me. Well, not *everything*. I actually have a lot more to say, but that will be for my next book...

But more importantly, you're now armed with the knowledge on anything and everything you can do to reverse aging. Whether it's skincare, devices, injectables, lasers, or surgeries; internal wellness, mental health, fashion, or physical health. It's all been laid out for you. Now, what will you do with it? The power to reverse your age (or in my case, *freeze* my age) lies in your own perfectly manicured hands!

If you opened this book in a sad state of mind, feeling like it was too late for you to turn back the clock, I hope you now know it's NEVER too late. I want you to feel enlightened and inspired. I also want you to know that you can always be just as beautiful on the outside as you are on the inside— no matter your age.

Go ahead and read this sentence a few times aloud to yourself: My life does not end when my skin starts to sag!

I'll admit one final secret here to you now that we're such close friends. When I started writing this book, I was, admittedly, a little nervous. I've done everything under the sun (well, not *under the sun!* More like, out of the sun!). Would people think I'm crazy? Would they make it halfway through the Introduction before losing hope that I'm not some sort of plastic pseudo-human walking around Miami Beach with my head in the clouds? Then, something happened. It felt so good to share everything with you, that it kept pouring out. I went back to each chapter again and again to add more. And that's exactly why it felt so important (and good!) to share my experiences—to have the truth out there so other woman aren't scared or embarrassed to do these things too.

It's likely that you're not going to do *everything* I've done (it really is like a freakin' full-time job keeping up, not to mention the costs!), but even using a few of the tactics we talked about will help. A tweak here and a tuck there can be a huge confidence boost! And remember, if you want some tweaks and adjustments—don't let anyone stop you! It's your life. And it's *your* body.

I'm sure by the time you've read this book, I've already tried a bunch of new tricks, and I look forward to sharing them with you. Let's stay in touch. If you haven't already, be sure to follow me on Instagram @SandraLenaSilverman for point of reference videos on everything you've learned in this book. And, if I'm trying a new procedure or new wellness tactic, I post it there, so you'll always be up to date. Feel free to DM me too—I welcome messages and I'd love to chat and get to know you! If you have questions, send them over, too…I'm here to help you! I'll be rounding up questions and doing regular Q&A sessions on Instagram.

I'll close on one last note. The real beauty in life comes from loving yourself, no matter what. Remember my life coach, Peter's, important message to speak kindly to yourself every day. If you take nothing else from this book, take that and run with it!

Here's to self-love and eternal youth!

About the Author

Sandra Lena Silverman is an author and Miami-based beauty and wellness advocate. In an effort to turn back the clock on aging, Sandra has tried every skincare product, treatment, procedure, and surgery. Now, she's eager to share her tried and true secrets for recapturing youth. Follow her on social: @SandraLenaSilverman.

About the Co-Author

Erica Florentine is the New York Times bestselling author of *Tremendous: The Life of a Comedy Savage*. Erica spent more than a decade working in journalism, public relations, and corporate communications. Her work has appeared in Huffington Post, Bustle, Thought Catalog, and WebMD.